D1423593

Pediatric Massage
REVISED
For the Child With Special Needs

Kathy Fleming Drehobl

B.S., OTR/L

Mary Gengler Fuhr

B.S., OTR/L

Foreword by

Rhoda Erhardt

M.S., OTR, FAOTA

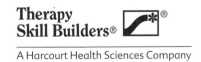

Therapy Skill Builders®

A Harcourt Health Sciences Company

Reproducing Pages From This Book

Many of the pages in this book can be reproduced for instructional or administrative use (not for resale). To protect your book, make a photocopy of each reproducible page. Then use that copy as a master for photocopying or other types of reproduction.

Library of Congress Cataloging-in-Publication Data

Drehobl, Kathy Fleming.
  Pediatric massage for the child with special needs / Kathy Fleming Drehobl, Mary Gengler Fuhr ; foreword by Rhoda Erhardt.—Rev.
      p. cm.
    Includes bibliographical references.
    ISBN 0-7616-4092-4 (pbk.)
    1. Massage for infants.
    2. Massage for children. I. Fuhr, Mary Gengler. II. Title.
RJ53.M35 D74 2000
615.8'22'083--dc21   00-008442

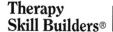
Portions of this work were published in previous editions.

0761640924

1 2 3 4 5 6 7 8 9 10 11 12 A B C D E

Printed in the United States of America.

Visit our website at www.tpcweb.com.

Dedication

This book is dedicated to the memory of Paula Tadano, M.Ed., C.H.T., OTR/L

Paula Tadano was a dear friend and colleague. Paula was the mother of two children, Daniel and Michael, as well as the spouse of her husband, Jim. She was an occupational therapist from Phoenix, Arizona who committed her life to helping people in her professional and personal life. Paula was an assistant professor at the Arizona School of Health Sciences. She was respected and honored by the faculty and students. Her committment to teaching and her compassion toward all made her presence a treasure. Her life was tragically taken by cancer in a short time during the authoring of this book. Although we will always miss her physical presence, her teachings will continue in our hearts. Thank you, Paula, for everything, but most of all for *touching* our hearts and minds.

About the Authors

Kathy Fleming Drehobl graduated from Indiana University with a B.S. degree in occupational therapy. She is currently practicing in the Phoenix, Arizona area and has practiced pediatric occupational therapy for 16 years. Kathy is certified in infant massage and myofacial release. Kathy has completed the 8-week basic neuro-developmental therapy (NDT) course as well as the advanced baby NDT course. She also has assisted in NDT courses.

Kathy has taught academically at the Arizona School of Health Sciences and clinically in workshops around the country. She was recently awarded the Distinguished Acheivement award through the Arizona OT association. She currently is pursuing a masters-doctoral program in computer technology in education. Kathy has worked with children and their families in hospitals, developmental centers, high-risk newborn follow up, private practice, public schools, and infant-stimulation programs.

Mary Gengler Fuhr graduated from the University of Wisconsin with a B.S. degree in occupational therapy. She has worked in pediatrics since 1982. She currently is in private practice in the Seattle, Washington area. Mary is a certified infant massage instructor. She has completed the 8-week basic Neuro-Developmental Treatment (NDT) course and the NDT baby course. Mary's background in sensory integration includes practicum coursework, as well as certification in the administration and interpretation of the Southern California Sensory Integration Tests and The Sensory Integration and Praxis Tests.

Mary has been an instructor in the Occupational Therapy Assistant Program at Green River Community College and has presented workshops around the country. She has had the opportunity to work with children and their families in developmental centers, public schools, Rosemary White's clinic, and private homes.

Acknowledgements

Writing this book has been an ongoing journey and the fulfillment of a dream for us. We have been committed to exploring, developing, and sharing the benefits of pediatric massage since we met in 1987. Throughout the process of presenting workshops and writing this book, we have benefited from the expertise and help of parents, children, and professionals from around the country. We are indebted to all of those who have offered their knowledge, skills, and enthusiasm to us. Massage for children with special needs continues to be a work in progress.

We are especially grateful to:

Our husbands Steve and *Bob, parents,* and *families* for their constant support and encouragement throughout both the ideation and creation of our workshop, video, and this book.

Our children Erik, Matthew, Michael, and *Emma* for their forbearance and unconditional love during the lengthy process of authoring this book. Sharing massage with our children has been a deeply enriching experience. They continue to inspire us to expand this work and keep us aware of the therapeutic value of touch in parenting.

Victoria Ryecroft, Cody Brown, Seth Rich, Katie Layzell, and *Trevor Barton* and *their families,* who shared their massage experiences in photographs so line art could be rendered.

Rhoda Erhardt, M.S., OTR, FAOTA, for her generosity, support, and encouragement of our work throughout the years and especially for her insightful contribution to this book.

Dr. Melvin Morse for his sensitivity to children's health and well-being and ongoing support of our infant massage projects.

Shereen Farber, Ph.D., OTR, FAOTA, who has shared her time, wisdom, and expertise in helping us integrate the world of caring touch with solid neurological principles.

Gay Lloyd Pinder, Ph.D., CCC-Sp, for sharing her time, self, and expertise in the area of oral motor development and treatment.

Marsha Dunn Klein, M.Ed., OTR, who gave invaluable encouragement with enthusiasm and kindness.

Rodd Hedlund, M.Ed., for providing us with excellent resources, information, and feedback about developmental care in the intensive care nursery, infant behavior, and early intervention.

Workshop participants who continually share their expertise and enrich our knowledge base.

The *Touch Research Institute* that has expanded the body of knowledge related to massage by expansive research with diverse populations. We support their work and look forward to their continued, admirable efforts in research.

Vimala Schneider McClure, a pioneer in the practice of infant massage in the United States, and the *International Association of Infant Massage* for providing inspiration for the development of this work.

Preface

As pediatric clinicians, we are constantly seeking methods of facilitating developmentally appropriate adaptive responses as well as promoting parent-infant interaction. Tactile intervention has long been a successful way to impact sensory systems. The authors would like to present this publication as a *guideline* to massage for children with special needs.

In this revision, we have included updated research, theory, and clinical information related to pediatric massage. Each chapter has been updated to reflect current literature and practice. Specifically, the Strokes chapter has been revised to include clinical implications. The Reference section also has been greatly expanded.

We hope these will assist practitioners and parents in safe and effective use of massage for children with special needs. We are confident that gentle touch and massage can be a positive and enjoyable experience for most children.

There are many excellent texts outlining massage strokes for children. The authors have chosen the strokes in this text because they:

- are easily adapted for children with special needs.
- can be used in conjunction with therapeutic positioning and handling
- help promote the attainment of therapeutic and educational goals
- enhance parent-child interaction
- have proved to be clinically valuable

A powerful sensory intervention, massage introduces many physical, social, and somatosensory benefits for children. This material is best used as a supplement to existing team-oriented therapeutic and educational programming. Massage is a holistic contribution to family-centered intervention and may be utilized by a variety of people involved in the child's program, including parents, therapists, educators, nursing staff, care providers, relatives, and friends.

As is always the case when children with special needs are involved, it is important to consult with medical personnel to assure that massage will be a safe and therapeutic intervention.

A Historical Perspective

Touch and massage have always been part of the human experience. Many cultures have offered insights into the therapeutic value of tactile intervention such as swaddling, skin-to-skin contact, and massage. The Eskimo culture has demonstrated the importance of swaddling in preservation of body temperature and promotion of calming behavior in infants. Medical personnel in Bogota, Columbia, have introduced the kangaroo care method of providing skin-to-skin contact for preterm infants. In this method, the undressed infant is placed between the mother's breasts, underneath her clothing, to promote feeding, body temperature regulation, and calming (Anderson, 1986). In recent years fathers also have been involved in providing this ventral-to-ventral, tactile input. In some regions of India, infants are regularly bathed and massaged with a variety of oils. These cultural influences and many others have helped shape the current use of gentle touch and massage with children.

Recent research with premature and term infants, as well as other populations with special needs, has led to the *rediscovery* of an ancient art to provide pleasurable touch to infants and children. The use of massage in pediatric care is further supported by clinical observations associated with the use of touch in therapeutic programming. The therapeutic benefits of touch/massage may range from parent-infant interaction to physiological changes. Touch and massage are done in many ways—swaddling; pressure; gliding strokes; gentle friction; or simple, sustained hand placement. This gives the massage giver conservative methods of providing tactile input to medically fragile children, as well as healthy, typically developing children.

We would like to see our culture embrace touch as essential for any child's health and well being. This revised edition expands on our initial observations and current knowledge about massage. Through our therapeutic interventions with children, teaching of workshops, and ongoing research, we have provided an updated, thorough resource to guide the massage giver toward the safe and therapeutic use of massage. We hope that massage will become a consistent, therapeutic interaction, and that children with special needs will be *touched* literally and emotionally. Kind, compassionate touch coupled with sound knowledge of massage principles is a powerful and therapeutic tool.

Foreword

The publication of this revised edition of *Pediatric Massage* could not be timelier. For more than 9 years since the first edition was written, it has been widely used by therapists, nurses, teachers, and parents to benefit children with special needs. During that time, there has been an explosion of interest and research in the fields of touch and massage, as well as more variety of accessible resources, such as web sites, books, music, and training programs, which are listed with addresses and phone numbers in the resource section. The authors have expanded this edition with new information gained not only from their many years of clinical experience and teaching but also from their perspective as parents, since each has a child with sensory integration issues. Their own children have especially enhanced their understanding of the significance of sensory input related to behavioral responses.

At a time when technology is escalating rapidly, it is essential for professionals to ensure that the art of healing is balanced with the science of healing. Emphasis continues to be placed on family centered care, and the role of massage in bonding and attachment has been expanded. The techniques so carefully described and illustrated are especially empowering for parents in creating successful interactions with their child.

Readers familiar with the first edition will find the organization and structure of the book unchanged, with new material inserted into the easily located chapters. For example, the chapter Potential Benefits of Massage now includes specific information for infants and children with colic, self-regulation disorders, sensory defensiveness, and autistic spectrum disorders, as well as children with spina bifida, congenital malformations, vision and/or hearing impairments, different types of cerebral palsy, terminal illness, and those affected by physical or drug abuse. Also, the chapter Getting Started now includes aromatherapy as part of the preparation process.

The research chapter has been updated with reported studies of the effects of massage on a greater variety of diagnoses, including cystic fibrosis, asthma, ADHD, dermatitis, diabetes, HIV, prematurity, and self-injurious behavior, as well as studies on typical preschoolers. Each abstract is summarized according to diagnosis, subjects, researchers, conditions, and results, giving the reader a birds'-eye view of each. In addition, the bibliography has been expanded and updated to include both current and historical listings of references relating to touch and massage.

The Massage Strokes chapter provides much more detail, adding specific clinical implications of each stroke. For example, one lower extremity stroke is done with the pattern of hair growth, thus producing inhibition or relaxation. It is useful and pleasurable for children with increased muscle tone since the pressure is very even and rhythmical. The stroke can be used therapeutically to elongate hamstring and adductor muscles, preparing for lower-extremity weight bearing. At the same time it promotes visual attention to the feet, assisting in downward gaze and convergence of eye muscles.

Detailed instructions and clear illustrations are provided to insure correct positioning, movements, and safety, and they are especially useful for teaching students and parents. It is with great enthusiasm that I recommend this practical manual as an outstanding source of information for all practitioners who recognize the value of the power of touch and the importance of its use as a clinical tool.

Rhoda P. Erhardt, M.S., OTR, FAOTA

Consultant in Pediatric Occupational Therapy

Maplewood, Minnesota

Contents

Chapter 4

Chapter 5

Chapter 6

Chapter 7

Chapter 8

Chapter 9

Chapter 10

Chapter 11

Chapter 12

Resources

References

Chapter 1

General Physiological Effects of Therapeutic Massage

Introduction

Adults who have received a massage know that it can relax the muscles and relieve stress, tension, pain, and stiffness. Conversely, massage can have an invigorating effect. The effects of massage vary from client to client as each person's specific needs differ. It is critical to have an understanding of a child's medical history and current status as well as a thorough assessment before beginning massage. It also is important to understand the physiological changes that can be produced by massage.

This book describes tactile intervention for children that differs from traditional adult massage (such as Swedish massage) in intensity, positioning, interaction, and goals. Pediatric massage is a powerful sensory tool that offers many benefits to children. It is a highly interactive experience with the massage giver carefully monitoring the child's responses and adjusting their intervention accordingly. This book was developed specifically for the purpose of introducing the benefits of massage to children with special needs in a safe, therapeutic, and pleasurable manner.

This chapter provides an overview of the general physiological benefits of massage, typically based on literature pertaining to adults. A detailed summary of the current research with children is provided in Chapter 8. Chapter 3 discusses specific benefits of massage for children with special needs based on clinical observations and experiences.

Massage benefits are objective and subjective. Fritz (1995) acknowledged that massage benefits must be measured by objective (observation) and subjective (client report) measures. She further elaborated that the global term *massage* might be quite varied in application. For instance, under the term *massage* are techniques such as Swedish massage, Indian massage, reflexology, and *shiatsu*. This makes it difficult to define the specific benefits of massage, as each technique offers different therapeutic value.

The Touch Research Institute at the University of Miami has made great strides in helping quantify and validate the efficacy and expansive benefits of massage. The institute's extensive research with infants, children, and adults has broadened our knowledge of the powerful therapeutic effects of massage.

Benefits

Massage increases and improves circulation—especially venous and lymphatic flow. According to Beck (1994), massage increases blood flow to the massaged area, enabling for better cellular nutrition and elimination. The increased blood flow occurring at a local level is accomplished by compression of soft tissues that empty venous beds and increases capillary blood flow (Fritz, 1995). An additional benefit is facilitation of the flow of venous blood and lymph back toward the heart for the process of elimination. Beck (1994) estimated that blood passes three times more rapidly through muscles being massaged than those at rest. Clinically, improved circulation is observed as healthy, pink, even skin coloration with an increase in skin temperature. Tappan (1998) suggested that regular use of massage in a health-care routine might reduce blood pressure and heart rate. In addition, she advocated the use of gravity as an assist to promote venous flow. Fritz (1995) concurred with the therapeutic use of gravity as well as range of motion to improve venous flow and return. Fritz also stated that circulation is improved primarily by biomechanical effects and secondarily through reflexive responses encouraging chemical secretions. She also related the importance that improved circulation offers in delivering nutrients and oxygen to local and general areas. Conversely, massage assists in eliminating carbon dioxide, metabolites, and other toxins. Effleurage strokes (long, sweeping, gliding strokes), moving from distal to proximal, particularly help in the movement of blood and lymph, clearing the interstitial spaces of metabolic wastes. This is important to optimize cellular nutrition and oxygenation (Newton, 1998).

Massage reduces certain types of edema. Edema occurs as a result of excess accumulation of fluid in the interstitial spaces. It often occurs in cases of immobility in which massage may prove therapeutic. Beck (1994) referred to edema as a circulatory abnormality that generally is described as puffiness in the extremities, with some cases being more widespread. Tappan (1998) discussed it not as a disease process but as a manifestation of altered physiological function. This may be mechanical or of a more serious nature such as protein imbalance, increased capillary permeability, or obstruction of lymph flow. Massage is **contraindicated** in the case of edema due to cardiac or kidney failure, torn tissues, internal bleeding, or the *pitted* type of edema. Refer to Chapter 7 for more information.

Massage improves skin nutrition and helps remove dry, scaly skin. Massage activates sensory receptors in the skin and increases the superficial circulation (Tappan, 1998). The friction associated with massage assists in removing dead skin. Moisture or lotion may facilitate this process. Tappan (1998) advocated the use of oil in massage where there is a dry climate, aging skin, or specific dry skin conditions. Natural oils from cold-pressed fruits and nuts are some of the best massage lubricants. It is important to consult with a dermatologist if there are skin allergies or fragility of the skin. Fernadez, Patkar, Chawla, Taskar, and Prabhu (1987) used corn oil in a study with preterm infants in India in an effort to preserve body temperature and provide nutrition. This study supports the therapeutic role of oils in massage.

Massage stimulates organs and body systems by reflex stimulation in the skin and subcutaneous tissues. Tappan (1998) described the reflex effects of massage as the result of pressure or movement in one part of the body having an effect on a different body part. She suggested that massage activates the sensory receptors of the skin and subcutaneous tissues, eliciting reflexive effects. This stimulation is passed along afferent (incoming) fibers of the peripheral nervous system directly to the spinal cord. From there it is possible that they disperse through central and autonomic pathways. Some examples may be capillary vasodilatation, vasoconstriction, or gooseflesh. There also may be potential sedation or stimulation of sensory reception with associated reduction or increase in pain. Massage must be monitored carefully to assure that these reflexive effects are therapeutic and do not produce undesirable effects. Some additional autonomic negative effects may include nausea, pallor, or sweating. The clinician should use massage so that desirable autonomic effects such as muscular relaxation, reduction of pain, and more focused attention may be produced. Fritz (1995) described some chemical reflexive responses associated with massage as being the secretion of endorphins and the release of histamine.

Field, et al. (1992) reported decreases in urinary cortisol (a stress hormone) and decreased norepinephrine levels as a result of massage, in a study of adolescents with depression. (Refer to Chapter 5 for more information about the tactile system's influence on the ANS.)

Massage prevents fibrosis/adhesions in muscles and decreases the tendency toward muscular atrophy and/or contractures. Beck (1994) described fibrosis as the process where muscle tissue is being replaced with fibrous connective tissue. Tappan (1998) referred to fibrosis as an abnormal collagenous connective tissue. Immobility, chronic stress, and trauma, as well as muscular/fascial restriction may contribute to this process. Massage may assist in restoring soft and connective tissue pliability and improve the performance of the tissue. Massage will not prevent atrophy in deneravated muscles; however, it may assist in recovery after injury if typical innervation is present (Tappan, 1988).

Massage maintains muscles in the best possible state of nutrition, flexibility, and vitality so that they can function at maximum potential. Typical muscles release metabolic waste products by milking toxins via the lymphatic and venous systems. As muscles relax, fresh blood flow brings necessary nutrients to the area. This balanced process may be disturbed through overactivity or underactivity of muscular contraction. In the overactive muscle, there may not be sufficient relaxation time for nutritive products to be produced. In addition, the muscle may become loaded with irritants and subsequently be denied of proper oxygen or become ischemic. Conversely, in the underactive muscle, the milking action may not be present to carry away irritant products. Massage may be effective in this case to enhance this process. It also may be a therapeutic strategy to restore or preserve soft tissue integrity, mobility, and muscular nutrition. This allows more opportunity for effective movement and function (Tappan, 1998).

Massage has been noted to decrease pain. Field, et al. (1997) reported significant decrease in the pain of patients with Juvenile Rheumatoid Arthritis. It is theorized that the pain is decreased secondary to stimulation of seratonin, a natural painkiller that is the base of many manufactured painkillers.

Field and her colleagues also studied massage in patients with burns, chronic fatigue syndrome, low-back pain, and fibromyalgia, resulting in significant pain reduction. The researchers hope that massage will compliment the use of drugs and minimize the need for potentially addictive narcotic medication.

Massage decreases anxiety, stress, and depression. Field, et al. (1992) discussed the role of massage in adolescents diagnosed with depression and adjustment disorder.

They discovered a decrease in cortisol, a hormone associated with stress. In addition they found less anxiety and stress behaviors when studying the role of massage with children who have asthma, atopic dermatitis, juvenile rheumatoid arthritis, cystic fibrosis, and diabetes. Field and her colleague's work continues to validate the psychological benefits produced by massage.

Massage may improve the general functioning of the immune system. Field and her colleagues (1992) continue to examine the role of massage in enhancing the immune system in patients with HIV and breast cancer. Additional studies in progress include pediatric oncology and prostate cancer (Cullen, et al., in preparation; Deiter, Field, Hernandez-Reif, in preparation).

Massage may contribute to general growth and development. The role of touch in growth and development has been historically documented in literature. Touch is vital to our well being, health, and relationships. Field, et al. (1986) has documented the role of massage in weight gain in pre-term infants. Massage also could be beneficial to children with failure-to-thrive syndrome. This must be confirmed through further research.

Summary

The physiological and psychological effects of massage may vary from child to child. The muscular, glandular, sensory, neurological, and vascular stimulation appears to benefit the body as a whole. As a beneficial part of a child's total health-care plan, massage offers enhanced physiological functioning and social-emotional growth.

Chapter 2

Psychosocial Considerations

Birth History

Pregnancy is a time of hope and expectation for most parents and families. All parents hope for an uncomplicated delivery and a happy, healthy baby. They spend hours developing a birth plan and discussing it with those who will be involved in the birth. Parents prepare for pregnancy by eating well; preparing their home for the infant; and educating themselves about pregnancy, delivery, and infant care. They buy, borrow, or make the items needed to welcome the newborn into their home. And they wait eagerly for the first touch and sight of their baby.

Sometimes, however, the events surrounding the birth do not occur as anticipated. Some babies are born very early or with a condition that makes medical care necessary. The newborn may be taken immediately from the mother and rushed to the intensive care nursery to save his or her life or to prevent further deterioration. The next few hours, days, weeks, or months may become an emotional roller coaster for the parents and family.

Parents who have lived through this trauma and separation have experienced many emotions. Initially, they may be fearful over the potential death of the baby, the mother, or both. It may be disconcerting to parents or family to see the infant attached by many wires to life saving equipment. Parents may wonder if they have caused the problems or could have prevented the situation. Mothers may feel that they have failed. They may have difficulty believing that the birth has occurred.

Parents often feel helpless and powerless about the health and developmental outcome of their baby. They may feel unable to protect their child. They may find themselves suddenly in a much more passive role in the care of their infant than they had envisioned. Some parents resent having to ask permission to touch, hold, or feed their baby. Time spent waiting for information about the infant's health status may seem endless. Medical information may be a confusing jumble of unfamiliar terminology.

Conversely, pregnancy may be a stressful time for some single mothers and two-parent families. Issues such as substance/physical abuse, poor prenatal care, financial difficulty, social challenges, and medical complications may contribute to a stressful pregnancy, delivery, and postpartum situation. These scenarios may make the bonding and attachment process complex and emotionally challenging. As early interventionists, clinicians have a unique opportunity to provide support and education to assist families in the bonding and attachment process. Massage is one of many tools that may facilitate this process and help families care for their child with special needs.

Parenting children with special needs may bring about a variety of emotional responses similar to the death and dying process described by Kubler-Ross (1993). This may be a cyclical process and come at various times for different families. A birthday may trigger grief if the child has not met milestones or skills as the parents had hoped. Gill (1997) is a parent of a child with Down syndrome who compiled quotes from parents of children with special needs in her publication, *Changed by a child.* One parent stated, "People always say to me, how did you survive it? But you don't have a choice, because you don't die" (p. 22).

Perske (1981) offered an excellent resource for parents of children with special needs titled, *Hope for the families.* He gave some simplified descriptions of how parents may feel. He described the *drags* as being run down and tired, the *speeds* as when you feel overwhelmed with so much to do, and the *blocks* as times when tough news comes from medical professionals and you feel the need to block it out. The *hurts* include a variety of behaviors that indicate the anguish and pain associated with having a child with a disability. Some may include restlessness, crying, or difficulty in sleeping. The *guilts* include when the parent blames himself or herself for the child's condition. The *greats* are moments when the parent may feel great about being a parent. This may follow a feeling of a few days ago that the parent was a horrible parent, yet the feeling of greatness is a much more pleasant alternative. The *hates* happen after hurting for a long time. The parent may search for a chance to blame anyone else for this difficult challenge. Finally there are the *escapes* when the parent feels the urge to flee and escape the situation.

Perske (1981) emphasized that each parent reacts differently and may feel none or all of these feelings. Many parents may have other feelings that can be added to this list. Perske offers some comforting strategies to assist parents through these stages. It is the authors' hope that massage can be a positive and therapeutic tool for the child and parent to work through during these challenging times.

Bonding and Attachment

Klaus, Kennel, and Klaus (1995) have extensively studied the area of bonding and attachment over the years. They used *bonding to* refer to the parent's emotional investment in their child. It is a process that builds and grows with repeated meaningful and pleasurable experiences. *Attachment,* on the other hand, is described as a tie that is developing from an infant toward his or her parents or caregivers.

They stress that from this initial emotional connection infants begin to develop a sense of themselves, enabling them to venture into their new world. Without this sense of themselves, children may not develop a sound sense of security and ability to trust.

Although immediate parent contact after delivery is an ideal situation for initiating the post-natal bonding process, (Klaus, Kennel, & Klaus, 1995) parents can become fully attached to their baby even if they lacked early contact, but the process may take more time. This is an important concept in that the bonding and attachment process may be disrupted with the medically fragile child or child with special needs. They recognized that initial bonding is not enough. The initial process of falling in love may be challenged as the demands of parenting increase, making staying in love more difficult.

Recognition of early contact has helped bring about hospital policies that increase the opportunity for parents to have private time with their healthy infant immediately following the delivery. Some hospitals encourage mothers and infants to stay together throughout the hospitalization instead of the traditional nursery arrangement. In addition, policies have been changed to assist parents in interacting with their fragile or premature infants. When the infant is medically stable, parents are encouraged to hold, feed, and interact with their infants. The concept of kangaroo care introduced in Bogata, Columbia, emphasized the importance of skin-to-skin touching in infants able to leave the isolette (Anderson, 1991). This method of skin-to-skin contact introduced having the unclothed infant lying on the mother's chest in order to enhance temperature regulation and promote breastfeeding. Although this concept was initially used with mothers exclusively, it is now being expanded to include fathers. The success of this program has made it more popular throughout the United States.

Klaus, Kennel, and Klaus (1995) recommended that when the premature infant has transitioned past the acute phase, both parents should touch and gently massage their baby. They reported a reduction in breath pauses, increased weight, and a shorter length of hospital stay. This touching should begin only upon the physician's approval.

The Role of Massage in Bonding and Attachment

Several components of the massage experience are thought to help facilitate attachment and bonding. According to McClure (1988) and Drehobl and Fuhr (1991), they include

- skin-to-skin contact
- eye-to-eye contact
- smiling
- soothing sounds

- cuddling
- smell
- response
- interaction

Skin-to-skin contact—*touch*—is one of the most important of these interactions. Mothers and fathers appear to have an innate desire to touch and hold their newborns. In a 1970 study by Klaus and associates, when undressed newborn infants were placed beside their mothers within hours of birth, the mothers began touching the babies' extremities with their fingertips. This touching progressed to massaging, with the mothers using their palmar surfaces to stroke the infants' trunks (Kennel & Klaus, 1982).

Body warmth also is a part of the touch experience. Many adults enjoy touching the softness and warmth of an infant's skin. Conversely, if the child is cold, the adult can provide body heat through skin-to-skin contact.

During massage, children often are cradled in their parents' laps, creating a face-to-face orientation. This *enface* position enhances the opportunity for eye contact between the child and the adult. In this position, children with visual impairments may center their heads or attend to the sound of their parents' voices.

The authors have observed an increase in children's vocalizations during massage, especially the chest massage. They have noted an increase in length of vocalization as well as the variety of sounds produced by children who rarely vocalize. The massage-giver has the opportunity to talk, sing, or make a variety of sounds to the child. This can shape the interaction into either a relaxing experience or playful game, depending on the individual's goals.

Many adults have noticed the distinctive smell of a newborn. Even a baby's clothing has a characteristic odor that may evoke pleasant memories. The olfactory system appears to be developed and discriminative during the newborn period. The close proximity of the child and adult during massage enables the exchange of body odors if unscented oil is used.

Turn taking is another process that occurs during the massage experience. The massage described in this book is unlike adult massage in that the recipient is encouraged to play a much more active role. Turn taking occurs when the child responds to the adult's voice, touch, and eye contact by producing sounds, looking or orienting, moving, smiling, or touching. The adult then reacts to the child's response, establishing a rhythm of communication. Parents and professionals can work together to identify the child's unique form of communication.

Summary

Many parents find that massage helps them feel closer to their children. Parents generally feel that massage is a successful interaction with their child, even when other home handling activities have been less positive. Massage also provides an opportunity for the parent to relax. It is human nature to repeat experiences that were satisfying and made us feel successful.

Chapter 3

Potential Benefits of Massage

Introduction

Massage is a useful sensory intervention that provides psychosocial and physiological benefits for a wide range of children with disabilities as well as typically developing children. It is an excellent adjunct to traditional therapy and educational programs. Massage provides benefits to the recipient and the giver. To achieve optimal results, massage techniques can be combined with therapeutic positioning/handling/dressing. The massage program is highly individualized according to the child's postural tone, reflex activity, behavior, modulation of sensory input, and the goals of the family.

The specific benefits described in this book are based on clinical observation and parent feedback, supplemented by information available in the literature. Research regarding the long-term effects of massage for infants and children is in progress. However, current literature relating to pediatric massage will be discussed in Chapter 8.

Common Benefits of Massage

Massage may enhance parent-child attachment and bonding. The *enface* position, with the child in supine, helps promote a positive social interaction. This position is preferred, if possible, because it enhances eye contact and parent interaction. Massage provides caregivers a unique opportunity to discover their child's specific preferences with soothing touch. This communication may assist in strengthening the parent-child bond. Chapter 2 describes components of massage that contribute to the attachment/bonding process.

Successful massage interactions may help increase parental confidence. Caregivers often relate that massage is a successful part of their home program. Some caregivers don't feel confident in their ability to adequately perform home handling and exercise techniques as recommended by their therapeutic team. The massage strokes are a natural extension of the caressing and rubbing used routinely at home. Caregivers derive satisfaction from using touch to elicit a pleasurable response from their child. They also are more likely to use an intervention consistently if they believe it is successful. Limited initial contact with a fragile infant may preclude initial confidence in handling. Massage serves as a positive introduction to loving touch.

Massage may help deepen respiration by mechanical assistance and the tactile system's effect upon the autonomic nervous system. Many neurologically involved children present with a highly elevated and flared rib cage with associated abdominal hypotonia that contributes to inefficient patterns of respiration. Massage may be used clinically to increase chest expansion (enabling the lungs to expand) and deepen inhalation and exhalation. The chest massage incorporates elongation of the pectoral and intercostal musculature. This may mechanically allow the rib cage to expand, producing a deeper respiratory cycle. This may be coordinated with inhalation and exhalation to further its therapeutic value. Neuro-developmental training specific to the respiration area is a valuable asset when using the chest massage.

The relaxation produced by the tactile system's influence on the parasympathetic nervous system also may help slow an elevated respiratory rate, thus improving the efficiency of breathing. Children with asthma may benefit from gentle stroking as a method of calming during an acute episode, and a full massage between episodes.

Massage may help improve blood and lymphatic circulation. Children with neuro-motor impairment often are challenged by gravity and display limited ability to assume antigravity positions. The quality and range of muscular contractions may not be sufficient to provide the pumping action necessary for adequate lymphatic drainage. Clinical signs of poor circulation may include webbing, mottling, or cyanosis of the hands and feet.

Massage, combined with antigravity positioning of extremities, enables gravity to help move fluid toward the heart. (Chapter 11 discusses positioning in more detail.) Swedish massage techniques involve firmly stroking extremities in a distal to proximal direction (i.e., from the hand to the shoulder). This combination of pressure and direction enhances the mechanical return of fluid toward the heart. The resulting effect is increased skin-surface temperature and even skin coloration with a slightly reddened response. Active movement will further enhance this circulation.

Massage may enhance awareness of body parts through visual, tactile, and proprioceptive input. Children with decreased antigravity movement and sensation may have limited opportunity to independently explore body parts. Extremities may appear *stuck* against the supporting surface, thereby inhibiting visual and tactile contact. This may be combined with tactile hypersensitivity or extremity neglect.

Visual contact with the lower extremities is extremely important for the development of visual convergence, midline head control, and downward visual gaze (Bly, 1994). This also is an opportune time to provide auditory input through the naming of body parts. Singing of children's songs or nursery rhymes often helps visual attention, language development, and vocalizations. Some songs (e.g., "This Little Piggy," "Head, Shoulders, Knees, and Toes," "Where is Thumbkin") can be coordinated with the strokes to promote recognition of body parts.

Massage provides symmetrical tactile input to both extremities. Use positioning with massage strokes to provide multi-sensory input to promote recognition of total body scheme. Many of the children in therapy programs lack the ability to spontaneously explore their body; thus, this intervention serves to assist in enhancing body awareness. Reaching for the hands, knees, legs, and feet is encouraged during the massage to emphasize antigravity control.

Massage may help reduce hypersensitivity to tactile input. As the massage progresses, the child may startle less or have a less aversive response to touch. Massage may be used for some children as an overall modulator of tactile input prior to the introduction of more specific tactile/proprioceptive techniques (i.e., oral motor stimulation). If the child is extremely sensitive, massage may need to be introduced gradually over a period of time. Slowly increasing the amount of tactile input may help the child successfully accommodate to the touch without becoming disorganized or agitated. Pressure is monitored carefully to assure a child's adaptive response. A goal of massage for the child with tactile defensiveness may include having the child more adaptively approach or accept tactile input. Massage is an excellent adjunct to provision of a sensory diet as advocated by Wilbarger and Wilbarger (1995).

Massage may increase the quality and quantity of phonation/vocalization. Face-to-face positioning enables optimal turn-taking opportunities. The massage giver encourages imitation of sounds, facial expressions, and words. The interaction paired with elongation to the pectoral and intercostals musculature further support the improved phonation. Increased variety and length of vocalization often are observed, especially during the chest massage. Massage also encourages children to use nonverbal and verbal communication in response to pleasurable strokes, and to express the desire for a stroke to be repeated. Speech and language pathologists provide excellent input in this area.

Massage may enhance gastrointestinal functioning. The underlying truncal hypotonia associated with some conditions, including cerebral palsy, Down syndrome, and spina bifida, make consistent elimination difficult. Abdominal massage may assist, both mechanically and reflexively, the movement of fecal matter through the large intestine. Massage may be used to aid the movement of contents through the large intestine (Beck, 1994). Children who tend to have difficulty relieving gas often benefit from massage to the abdomen.

Massage may provide general relaxation for the caregiver and child. It often may be stressful and time-consuming to care for children, particularly if they have extraordinary needs. Parents need a time when they can relax or be playful with their child. The massage experience provides a time when parent and child can relax together. Field, Hernadez-Reif, Quintino, Schanberg, and Kuhn (1998) reported that in a program where grandparent volunteers massaged infants in the NICU, the massage givers benefited as well as the infants. Those benefits included decreased anxiety, improved mood, depressed cortisol, and a better lifestyle as evidenced by fewer doctor visits and increased social contacts.

The Child With Hypertonicity

The term *muscle tone* refers generally to the tone in the resting state of a muscle (Brodal, 1998). In neuromotor damage, there often is an increase or decrease in postural tone referred to as either hypertonicity or hypotonicity. The next two sections will address general definitions and indications for massage for children with these conditions.

Hypertonicity refers to a state of increased postural muscle tone despite attempts to relax (Brodal, 1998). Bly (1983) emphasized the concept of *fixing* as a child's strategy to achieve postural alignment against gravity. *Fixing* often occurs in muscles historically thought to be spastic, such as the adductors, hamstrings, and biceps. Current literature suggests that hypertonicity may have its etiology in initial fixing, and over time as the improper patterns are repeated, the intrinsic or viscoelastic properties of the muscle may change (Brodal, 1998). Clinically, children with hypertonicity present with stiffness with difficulty moving efficiently against gravity.

Some of the diagnoses commonly characterized by hypertonicity are

- spastic diplegia,

- spastic quadriplegia,

- some hemiplegias,

- traumatic head injury, and

- near-drowning.

Use slow, rhythmic, stroking when working with children with hypertonicity.

Massage may assist in increasing a child's functional mobility by relaxation of the muscles, improved circulation, and increased available range of motion. Active movement is encouraged throughout the massage. Combined with therapeutic handling and movement, massage may produce significant gains in overall mobility and function. The tactile system's influence on the autonomic nervous system (ANS) also serves to reduce tone. (See Chapter 5 for more information on the ANS). Tonal change associated with massage can appear as decreases in shoulder elevation, scapular retraction, hand fisting, and an overall relaxed posture.

Massage may facilitate lip closure and decrease the tendency for cheek and lip retraction. Therapeutic handling and positioning during massage may lead to overall tonal reduction in the hypertonic child. The strokes providing direct tactile input to the face move in a direction that facilitates lip closure. Jaw control and cervical alignment are provided, if necessary, to assure proper alignment of the mouth for these strokes.

Massage offers an opportunity to elongate specific muscle groups. Throughout the massage, experienced therapists may use specific techniques that elongate certain muscle groups such as the pectorals, obliques, hamstrings, and heelcords. It is important to combine this with functional movement and play to derive optimal benefits. Experienced therapists may incorporate massage with other soft tissue or mobilization techniques in which they have been properly trained.

Massage may be used as a preparation for movement. Massage is an excellent way to introduce touch from the therapist before facilitating movement in a treatment session.

The Child With Hypotonicity

Hypotonicity is low muscle tone ranging from complete lack of tonic control to slight hyperextensibility of soft tissues. Clinically, children with hypotonicity present with floppiness and hypermobility. They, too, are limited in moving against gravity due to low muscle tone. They may use a wide base of support in sitting and standing to become more stable.

Conditions involving hypotonicity may include

- Down syndrome

- congenital hypotonicity

- cerebral palsy—hypotonia

Use more brisk, arrhythmic stroking when massaging the child with hypotonicity.

Massage may help promote activation of the musculature of the proximal joints. The pressure, rate, rhythm, and direction of stroking may be modified to facilitate tone and proximal stability. Antigravity reaching is encouraged as well as midline alignment of the upper and lower extremities. *Massage is not always used for relaxation—it can be a useful tool to promote tone and arousal in the child with hypotonicity.* The experienced therapist may combine the use of massage with treatment techniques such as joint compression or slight traction to facilitate proximal control. Joint compression may be introduced with the Swedish stroking (proximal direction); traction may be used with the Indian stroking (distal stroking). For a description of strokes, see Chapter 12. Regi Boehme's reference materials (as listed in the References) describe specific uses of compression and traction. It is important to note the integrity of the joint structure in the child with hypotonicity—subluxation may occur if an inappropriate amount of traction is used.

Massage may help promote an appropriate level of arousal in the noninteractive/lethargic child. A primary goal of massage is to elicit interaction and focusing behaviors. The quiet alert state is ideal for learning and interaction. (Chapter 4 discusses state behavior in detail.) Because the child is not hungry, fatigued, or irritable, he or she is best able to benefit from sensory and social stimulation.

The massage goal is to help the child with lethargy move toward a more organized state—one in which the child processes environmental information most efficiently. Modify the environment, strokes, and positioning to encourage optimal eye contact, interaction, and orientation to the surroundings. Brisk music, added vocal inflection, and perhaps an increase in visual stimulation can help produce a more animated environment.

Massage promotes orientation of extremities toward midline. Therapeutic positioning is used to assist the child in antigravity control. The interventionist holds the extremities in a position that promotes visual and tactile contact with extremities—the feet and hands. (Chapter 11 discusses positioning in more detail.)

Massage may be used to promote lip closure. To promote oral closure, the face strokes in this book have been adapted to proceed toward midline. This may be useful as a preparation for feeding. Jaw control and cervical alignment also are, if necessary, used to optimize the alignment of the oral mechanism.

The Child With Spina Bifida

Combine massage with early home handling techniques/positioning to minimize deformity, maintain skin integrity, promote circulation, enhance existing sensation, and provide visual awareness of the lower extremities. Traditional range-of-motion exercises also can be combined with massage strokes.

With medical supervision, massage also can be coordinated with bowel elimination programs. Massage can be a pleasant alternative to suppositories or rectal stimulation. In some cases, bladder catheterization may be necessary before massage. As with other issues of elimination, the interventionist should consult with a physician to rule out structural problems.

The Infant With Colic

The terms *colic* and *high need* often are used interchangeably. In the literature, most authorities agree that colicky infants share the following symptoms or behaviors (Jones, 1992; Scheider, 1989; Sears, 1991).

Excessive crying. This often is characterized by an infant who cries in excess of three hours a day, particularly during the evening. These infants lack the ability to console themselves and frequently are inconsolable by the caregiver. The cry has a frantic quality and is high-pitched or shrill.

Extreme sensitivity. Many infants with colic appear to be hypersensitive to environmental stimuli. These infants often startle easily to stimuli such as a sneeze or a flicker of light coming through their room. Some theorists feel that the infant with colic also has a heightened sensitivity to internal stimuli. Some, for example, become agitated by the sound of their rumbling stomachs.

Colicky body language. Many caregivers have described postures such as arching of the back and flailing of the extremities, sometimes alternating with legs drawing up very tightly into the abdomen. These postures often discourage caregivers from the cuddling that is so important in the bonding process.

The appearance of abdominal pain. Many parents of irritable infants state that the crying often is associated with gastric distention and pain, legs drawn into the abdomen, and intense high-pitched cries. Some infants have frequent constipation and/or associated retention of gas.

Infants with colic may be generally described as requiring more than average infant care. Caregivers often describe their infants as intense, demanding, draining, uncuddly, and unpredictable. Infants displaying these characteristics typically are younger than 2 months to 3 months of age. If these symptoms last longer than 6 months, they are referred to as disorders of self-regulation and have a correlation with potential developmental problems (DeGangi, 1991).

Many clinicians and caregivers have reported that abdominal massage in combination with an appropriate diet have significantly reduced gas-related *colic* in some children. Combined with a program to reduce or filter environmental stimuli, massage can provide a soothing sensory experience that may assist the child in calming.

Caregivers need a great deal of support and sensitivity from therapists and others during this difficult time in their child's development. Assist caregivers with relaxation strategies before beginning the massage. Massage can boost the caregivers' confidence by giving them a consistent method to console their child or lower the child's state. Be sure to consult with a physician before initiating massage with a child with colic. There may be an organic etiology responsible for the colic or irritability that may be aggravated by massage.

The Child With Self-Regulatory Disorders

DeGangi (1991) described self-regulatory disorders as persistent symptoms lasting beyond 6 months of age and related to four areas:

- arousal,
- feeding,
- sleep, and
- behavior.

Caring for these children may prove very challenging and exhausting. Massage offers relaxation for the caregiver and child, as well as a consistent method of consolation. Massage also may assist in modulation of sleep/awake states. Including massage as a part of the child's sensory diet may lessen behavioral irritability.

The Child With Sensory Defensiveness

Sensory defensiveness has been described as a continuum of approach and avoidance behaviors (Wilbarger & Wilbarger, 1991). Sensory defensiveness encompasses multiple sensations such as tactile, oral, auditory, visual, and vestibular. Children with sensory defensiveness may respond adversely to sensations typically integrated by other individuals. For example, simple tags or seams on clothing are largely unnoticed by most people, yet a child with sensory defensiveness may be highly aware and irritated by this sensation.

Many sensory adaptations need to be made for these children to be successful. Wilbarger and Wilbarger (1991) described the therapeutic use of sensory diet. As with the need for a nutritional diet, they explained that people need a steady sensory diet to maintain their arousal, attention, and adaptive behavior. Wilbarger and Wilbarger advocate the use of a brushing technique followed by proprioception to the joints. This technique is supplemented throughout the day with other sensory media to assist the child in modulating sensory input. Massage may assist the child with sensory defensiveness in modulation of sensory input, producing more adaptive behavior (i.e., greater flexibility, less fight-or-flight behavior, reduced stress). It can be a helpful component of the sensory diet when used regularly.

It can be an exhausting process to carefully monitor the child's sensory diet, yet being proactive certainly helps during transition times. Children with sensory defensiveness are often unpredictable in their response to specific sensory stimuli. For instance, in one environment light touch may not bother them, whereas in another environment, such as school, they may perceive the stimulus as aversive. Sometimes this is associated with behavioral outbursts presenting parenting and school management challenges. Although the massage giver or caregiver cannot control the child's entire sensory environment, the massage giver or caregiver knows the child will be more successful and happy if certain sensations are provided or avoided as a part of the daily routine. Routine and structure may be necessary throughout the child's development; however, as the child matures and becomes aware of sensory sensitivities, the symptoms of sensory defensiveness improve over time. Massage has been an integral part of the authors' children's sensory diet since infancy. They ask for this input along with aromatherapy, vibration, and deep pressure to keep them calm and behaviorally organized. Massage is a powerful tool in helping reduce sensory defensiveness and enabling the child to cope more effectively in varying environments.

The Child With Terminal Illness

In the case of terminal illness, massage may be used to comfort the child. Caregivers also may find that massage affords a special time to interact with the child and provide pleasurable input. This is particularly important to the child who is experiencing painful medical procedures and may associate touching with stress or pain. The intimate experience of massage also may assist caregivers in the grieving process.

Some medical conditions, such as cardiac conditions or cancer in an active state, might be aggravated by the stroking of massage. Consult with the child's physician. An alternative is to place a relaxed hand gently on the abdomen, back, or head. For more information about medical considerations, refer to Chapter 7.

The Child With Autistic Spectrum Disorder

Autism is a spectrum disorder in which the symptoms and characteristics can present themselves in a wide variety of combinations and with varying severity. Autism impacts the typical development of the brain in the areas of social interaction and communication skills. People with autism have difficulties in verbal and non-verbal communication, social interactions, and leisure or play activities. They also may exhibit repeated body movements (e.g., hand flapping, rocking), unusual responses to people, attachment to objects, perseveration, aggression, and difficulty with transitions or changes in routine. Children with autism may be overreactive to many sensory inputs such as sound, light, light touch, smell, food textures and tastes, and movement. They may crave others such as deep pressure or spinning. The abilities of a child with autism may fluctuate because of difficulties in processing, attention, or anxiety. People with autism have a unique perspective of the world.

Several related disorders are grouped under the broad heading of Pervasive Developmental Disorder (PDD) and are characterized by severe and pervasive impairment in several developmental areas (Autism Society of America Home Page, November 1999).

Many children with autism and PDD can have positive outcomes when given family support, early intervention, behavioral intervention, structure, and an appropriate sensory diet.

Massage and aromatherapy may assist the child with autism or PDD in calming and reducing anxiety in stressful situations. Improved eye contact, vocalization, and attention also may be observed during or after massage, which can be offered in conjunction with deep pressure from large pillows or bean bags, or vestibular input such as swinging in a hammock or a platform swing.

The Child With Congenital Malformations

Massage may be a tool to facilitate pleasurable tactile input for the child with congenital malformations. Joint limitations or deformities may interfere with the child's ability to initiate tactile experiences independently. Caregivers also may be reluctant to stroke extremities that appear or *feel* unusual. Massage also may assist the child in body awareness and accepting the uniqueness of his or her body.

Massage may provide a way to facilitate the bonding/attachment process. Massage was introduced to a child diagnosed with metatrophic dwarfism. Therapeutic goals included increasing range of motion and facilitating active movement and functional hand play. Massage was introduced in hopes of establishing parent-child bonding/attachment, providing pleasurable tactile input, preparing the child for range of motion and helping the parents accept the child's body structure. Smiles and vocal exchanges showed that the child immensely enjoyed the experience. Massage became a daily routine for the family and part of the home nursing care plan.

The Child With Visual Impairment

Massage is an excellent way to interact with the child who is blind or visually impaired. Touch can enhance the child's feelings of security. It may help the child form meaningful associations with sounds, smells, and sensations. Touch may help prevent a visually impaired or blind baby from withdrawing from the outside world. Touch can be a way of supporting the infant or child's curiosity and desire to explore and participate in their environment (Harrell, 1984).

Harrell (1984) makes recommendations for working with blind and visually impaired children. The suggestions, which can easily be incorporated into the massage routine, include:

For babies

- Speak to the baby by name. This lets the baby know that he or she will be part of the process.

- Talk to the baby. Your intonation helps develop a relationship. Assist the baby in learning to anticipate changes by talking before touching or moving him or her.

- Describe the body parts you touch and gently massage. Touching and stroking are pleasurable and help the baby develop a body image.

- Hold and cuddle the baby frequently.

- Observe the reactions of the baby's entire body to determine responsivity.

For young children

- Address the child by name and introduce yourself by name. You may pair your name with a gentle touch to the child's leg or other body part. Consistently touch the same place each time you identify yourself so that the child learns to associate you with that touch.

- Explain what you are doing. ("I'm putting oil in my hands. Now I'm rubbing my hands together.") Also explain what you will do next ("Now I will rub your leg").

- Name/describe the part of the body as you massage it.

- Let the child touch and explore the objects and materials you are using (such as the oil bottle, your hand, bath mitt, and positioning devices).

Other suggestions

- Make sure your voice reflects calmness and security.

- Decrease extraneous environmental sounds so that the child can concentrate on your voice, the sound of oil swishing, and the feeling of your touch. It's best *not* to use music until the child has developed a trusting relationship with you and the massage has become routine.

- Emphasize some of the sounds in the massage process, such as shaking the bottle of oil before opening it, or rubbing your hands together.

- A lightly scented natural oil will give the child additional information through the sense of smell.

- Make sure the child is positioned comfortably and securely. Adjust the lighting to the child's needs.

- Develop a massage routine. Always begin with the same body part and follow the same sequence of strokes. Additionally, in a preschool type of environment, have massage occur at a predictable time of the day. The use of aromatherapy will assist the child in identification and awareness of caregivers/teachers.

The Child With Hearing Impairment

In this case, it is crucial to maintain eye contact and provide the child with many visual cues. Initially, the massage giver or caregiver may want to choose only strokes that enable the child to maintain eye contact. (Some children with hearing impairments also have visual impairments. Explain or demonstrate the position and strokes to the child if moving him or her to a position without visual contact. The use of a lightly scented oil would give the child additional sensory input to compensate for the visual or auditory cues.)

To prepare the older child, first demonstrate the strokes on another child or a doll, or have the child look at pictures of a child being massaged. Sign language should be used in conjunction with verbal explanation throughout the massage.

The Preterm Infant

Caution: Consult a physician before beginning massage with premature infants because of their fragile status.

Many professionals and theorists have explored the benefits of massage for preterm infants. These studies differ immensely in type of stroking, duration of strokes, criteria measured, and health status of the infant. Chapter 8 compares and contrasts tactile research conducted with the premature population, and more information about the preterm population is in Chapter 6.

The interventionist or parent using massage with the premature population must proceed conservatively, bearing in mind the infant's fragile medical status. The premature infant's capacity to process tactile input is limited by a small surface area, immaturity, and the possible presence of medical conditions. Introduce strokes gradually, carefully monitoring the child's physiological and behavioral cues.

It also is important to monitor the infant's response after the input, as rebound phenomena may occur. If the infant receives too much stimulation, his or her body might have to work harder to restore the delicate premature homeostasis.

Neonatal intensive care unit (NICU) staffs throughout the country are working hard to reduce infant stress in the NICU environment. However, many medical procedures produce pain or discomfort in the infant. Massage offers a pleasant alternative to painful touch. If massage proves overstimulating, a gentle hand placement may help the infant relax.

A massage program for the premature infant may include goals such as

- reducing tactile sensitivity,
- assisting in modulation of extreme irritability,
- preparing for range of motion,
- providing calming-pleasurable tactile input,
- facilitating positive interaction between infant and caregiver, and
- promoting developmentally appropriate adaptive responses, such as hands to the mouth and tuck posture.

A physical therapist who attended a Pediatric Massage workshop allowed the speakers to massage her twins who were born prematurely. While her twins were in the NICU, she used kangaroo care with her babies, but said that she "would love to have been able to *do* something else with my boys . . . being a parent of babies in the NICU is a very difficult thing, and having PT/OT intervention would have been wonderful."

She wrote that after her twins experienced the massage during the workshop, they "slept so deeply on the way home and then at home. After their next feeding, Grandma was holding K., and she said that he was the most interactive she has ever seen him—and she sees the boys an average of once a week."

Infants Affected by Maternal Drug Abuse

The number of infants affected by maternal substance abuse has risen dramatically in recent years. Characteristics of these babies vary, but they often present with some of the following symptoms:

- prematurity
- low birth weight
- apnea
- seizures
- poor feeding skills
- poor state regulation
- increased or decreased tone
- poor visual tracking

- irritability
- excessive crying
- tremors
- disorganization
- difficulty with transitions
- poor interactive skills
- excessive motor activity
- delayed development

These characteristics often make caring for the infant difficult and frustrating. There may be a disruption of the bonding/attachment process because these babies often are difficult to console, less cuddly, and less alert or interactive.

Techniques currently used with this population tend to be inhibitory, aimed at consoling the baby and facilitating self-consoling. Hyde and Trautman (1989) identify several treatment techniques, including

- vestibular input for calming or alerting,
- deep touch/proprioception for calming and organizing,
- facilitation of flexion to assist with calming and central nervous system organization, and
- facilitation of oral skills.

Massage may be beneficial when used with the following guidelines adapted from the work of Kathleen A. VandenBerg (1990). VandenBerg, a specialist in the Neonatal and Developmental Medicine division at the Stanford University School of Medicine, is a leading expert in the area of prevention, identification, and management of agitation. She has developed a minimal-handling protocol and methods for avoiding stress in the

NICU. These methods also can be used with the drug-affected baby living in a home environment or therapeutic foster care situation.

- Massage the baby at the same time each day. Introduce new body parts to massage slowly to enable the child to sufficiently adapt to the input. Using the same sequence will further help in keeping a consistent, predictable routine throughout the massage.

- Allow the child to achieve a calm state before the massage. The baby also should be calm after the massage, before introducing the caregiving events.

- Provide the opportunity for sucking and grasping as a calming method during the massage.

- Provide an environment in which the child is protected from light and noise.

- You may need to wrap or swaddle parts or all of the baby's body to provide containment. Positioning with rolled-up blankets or foam cutouts around the body to maintain containment also may be useful. You initially may need to give deep-pressure touch/massage through the blanket in which the child is wrapped. Holding the hands or feet may be the initial acceptable level of tactile intervention for some infants.

- Prone or sidelying positioning is recommended as part of VandenBerg's minimal-handling protocol. Massage or tactile intervention such as holding the feet and hands can easily be done in either of these positions.

Further work and research will determine which strategies are most successful in the long-term social, emotional, cognitive, language, and motor development of the drug-affected baby. Massage is expected to play a key role in the treatment of these children.

The Physically Abused Child

Some people feel that massage can help abused children learn about *good touch*. However, be extremely sensitive when working with children who have been abused. A sense of trust must be developed. The person giving the massage needs to be exceptionally responsive to the child's verbal cues and body language. Counselors working with the child and family should be consulted before a massage program is begun to determine if it is appropriate. Ongoing communication with the counselors about the child's response is advised.

Once it is determined that massage is appropriate, there are some suggestions for working with a child who has been abused.

- Do not massage over blue or purple bruises, scratches, or open wounds. (See Chapter 7.)

- Massage may need to be introduced slowly, beginning with a simple hand placement on the back. Stroking may initially need to be limited to areas that the child perceives as *safe,* such as the back, lower legs, or feet.

- Some children feel more comfortable if they are clothed during the massage.

- The child should be in a position so as to feel in control. The child may prefer to sit, as opposed to lying down.

- In massaging most children, the adult raises his or her hands to help the child anticipate the massage. This should be *avoided* with the child who has been physically abused—it may be perceived as threatening.

The person introducing the massage program also needs to be sensitive to the *caregivers'* comfort level and experience with touch. One instructor had an enlightening experience when teaching an introductory infant-massage class to a group of single mothers attending an alternative high school.

Several of the young women seemed disturbed after viewing a videotape of beneficial massage situations. "I did not like the way that father was touching his daughter," said one young woman. Another asked, "How would the baby know if he or she were being massaged or molested?" After the class, the instructor was informed that many of the students in this class had been sexually abused.

Other Situations

Pre-casting. Massage can decrease hypersensitivity and fear before casting procedures. It also may be used to achieve increased joint range of motion in the extremity to be casted.

Post-surgical. One physical therapist reported using massage to reintroduce touch after surgery. He reported that after the surgery, the child was extremely fearful of health care professionals and therapy procedures. Massage helped gain the child's trust and reduce fear. After a few sessions, the child was more receptive to therapeutic handling.

Brachial plexus injury. Massage may be used to promote sensory recognition of the extremity and discourage the extremity disregard present in many children. Strokes may be combined with range of motion, positioning, and exercise as a part of a total therapy program.

Foster care placement/new adoption. Massage can help the child's transition to a new environment. Soothing strokes can provide comfort, establish rapport, and strengthen the relationship between the child and the foster or adoptive parents. To establish continuity of care, massage also may become part of the daily routine. If the child presents with special needs, adapted strokes can help achieve therapeutic goals. Massage therapy greatly assisted a family in bonding with a new child and getting to know his handling likes and dislikes. In the early stages of parenting, it provided a unique opportunity to express caring touch and welcome him into the family. Massage remains a part of the family routine even as he becomes older.

Before and after application of ankle/foot orthoses (AFOs) or standing in a prone stander, flexistander, or supine stander. Massage may decrease sensitivity and prepare the child for wearing orthoses and weight bearing through the lower extremities. Massage also can be used after removing AFOs to remove dead skin, enhance circulation, and provide warm human touch to areas that have been encased in plastic.

See Chapter 8 for a comprehensive review of current research on massage of infants and children with other diagnoses.

Chapter 4

Infant States

Introduction

How we feel greatly affects the way we interpret and respond to information in our environment. A touch that is pleasurable when we are well rested, healthy, and nourished may feel entirely different if we are stressed, exhausted, or ill. A child's response to massage will be influenced by the child's sleep/wake state at the time tactile intervention is introduced.

Kathryn Barnard, R.N., Ph.D., and Susan Blackburn, R.N., M.N., and their associates have worked extensively in the area of identifying infant states and their components and implications for care giving. A goal of their research, which culminated in the *Nursing Child Assessment Satellite Training* (NCAST) project, is to disseminate this information to those who work with families with infants and young children. For more information about this project, see Resources at the end of the text.

Definitions

In the NCAST Resource Manual, Blackburn (1989) defined a state as a cluster of characteristics that occur regularly together. The characteristics of individual states may include body activity, eye movements, breathing patterns, and type of response to external and internal stimuli.

The NCAST material identifies six infant states as

- deep sleep
- light sleep
- drowsy
- quiet alert
- active alert
- crying

The infant also may display brief transitional periods during which characteristics of more than one state may occur. Internal and external factors that may affect the infant's state include hunger, fatigue, noise, positioning, and handling (Blackburn, 1989). *State organization* "implies the ability to remain in a well-defined state for significant periods of time, and the smoothness of transition from one state to the nest" (Gunzenhauser, 1987).

Klaus, Kennel, and Klaus (1995) reported that for the first 45 minutes of life, babies are predominantly in the quiet alert state with their eyes in a wide gaze and opened brightly in a dimly lit room. This would demonstrate the amazing ability of the term infant to interact with his or her parents in the first moments of life.

The following table identifies the states and their qualities, and shows the most appropriate states for the introduction of massage.

State and the Introduction of Massage

Most infants tend to move smoothly between states. According to Blackburn (1989), "In each state, infants respond in a unique and predictable manner, not chaotically, but in an organized pattern. Infants use their states to control how much and what kind of input they receive from their environment." "Effective interventions should be aimed at facilitating the infant's control of state organization" (Gunzenhauser, 1987).

Generally, it is ideal to begin the massage when the infant is in the *quiet alert* state. The infant in this state is attentive and ready to interact with the caregiver, providing feedback to what is pleasurable. Communication between the adult and the infant in the quiet alert state is the most successful.

It is not realistic to expect a child to always be in the ideal state during scheduled treatment sessions. Many children with neurological dysfunction seem to experience extreme state disorganization—they appear to have difficulty remaining in a clearly defined state and shifting smoothly from one state to another. Some children, for example, spend an inordinate amount of time crying or sleeping; seldom do they experience the quiet alert state for any extended period of time.

In these situations, you may need to begin the massage with the child in an alternate state (preferably, the drowsy or active alert state), with the goal being to help the child achieve the quiet alert state. You may promote arousal in the drowsy or lightly sleeping child by providing brisk, but gentle, arrhythmical strokes.

Blackburn (1989) provides other ways to help the infant attain a more alert state, including:

- talking to the infant in a voice that varies in pitch and tempo,
- showing your face to the infant, and
- placing the infant in an upright position.

Note: Closely monitor the child with central nervous system dysfunction—some of these techniques may be overstimulating.

Conversely, slow, rhythmical strokes may help move an infant from the active alert to the quiet alert state, where better interaction can occur. For some infants a soothing voice, swaddling, use of a pacifier, or rocking may help the infant attain a calmer state (Barnard, 1989). Parents may find that these same techniques help the child move to a sleep state.

Some infants spend an excessive amount of time in the deep sleep state, with minimal awake moments for interaction. The infant in deep sleep will not be interactive with the caregiver. Massage is generally not recommended at this time. In rare cases where the infant is extremely sensitive to tactile input, gentle deep pressure or rhythmical

Infant States and Massage

	Deep Sleep	Light Sleep	Drowsy	Quiet Alert	Active Alert	Crying
Movement of body	Almost still May startle/twitch	Some movement	Variable activity level Generally smooth with mild startles	Little or much movement	Much movement May fuss	Much movement Color changes
Eyes	No movement	Eyelids flutter Rapid eye movement	Open and closed Heavy, dull, glazed	Open, bright, wide	Open, less bright	Tightly closed or open
Face	None except sucking bursts at regular intervals	May suck/smile May fuss briefly	May have some movements	Bright and shiny Focuses	Not as bright May fuss	Grimaces Cries
Breathing	Regular	Irregular	Irregular	Regular	Irregular	More irregular
Responsivity	Minimal, aroused only by very intense stimuli	More responsive than in deep sleep State may change	Delayed response State often changes	Most attentive	More sensitive to disturbing internal or external stimuli	Very responsive to unpleasant internal or external stimuli
Massage	Not recommended Begin only if child is extremely sensitive to tactile input and will not tolerate it in a higher state Not much feedback or interaction with caregiver	Brisk, arrhythmical strokes may arouse to quiet alert state Slow, rhythmical strokes may facilitate sleep		Ideal	Slow, rhythmical strokes may calm and lower state	Stop or modify massage

Adapted with permission from *Nursing Child Assessment Satellite Training Resource Manual*, NCAST Publications, 1989, University of Washington School of Nursing, Seattle, Washington.

stroking may be tolerated only in deep sleep. The goal here is to increase the child's acceptance of tactile input in states of greater consciousness/alertness.

Crying

The crying state is obvious to most observers. The reason for the crying may be harder to determine. This may be particularly true for children with neurological dysfunction.

Blackburn (1989) referred to crying as the infant's primary communication signal. It is a response to unpleasant internal or external stimuli. Internal stimuli may include fatigue or hunger; external stimuli may include cold temperatures or loud noises. Crying is an indication that the infant has reached his or her limit. Sometimes, infants are able to console themselves. However, they may need assistance from caregivers to return to a lower state.

Described here are the typical crying behaviors and some underlying causes (Jones, 1992; Scheider, 1989; Sears, 1991; Sears & Sears, 1996).

Hunger. A hunger cry is typically rhythmical, short, and explosive, followed by a breath-catching pause. The pause may be adaptive, as it allows the caregiver a chance to provide a breast or a bottle-feeding. Accompanying behavior may include sucking a fist or fingers for oral stimulation. If left unattended, the explosive cry may turn into a more intense pain or anger cry.

Sleepiness. This cry is less rhythmical than hunger or pain cries. It may be simply described as fussing. The baby may try to self-console by batting his or her ears, touching his or her hair, or sucking his or her fingers. The baby may rub his or her eyes or have the appearance of red eyes. He or she will not want to engage in play and may turn away from adults.

Thirst. This may appear the same as a hunger cry, with the infant being unsatisfied by formula. Jones (1992) related that infant formula may have an elevated sodium content and the infant may be thirsty. Individuals living in warm weather also may experience a thirst-oriented cry. One should, however, check with the child's pediatrician before introducing water, especially for young infants.

Internal Pain. Cries of pain typically have a sudden onset, reach a high pitch quickly, and stay at that pitch for a long duration. This is followed by a long pause, as if the infant is holding his or her breath. An alarming scream may follow the pause. The tongue may arch and the mouth may open wide. The chin, feet, and hands may quiver. Possible causes for this cry include gas, muscle aches, and allergic reactions.

Extremities may be drawn up or cycle tensely, sometimes accompanied by hand fisting. Facial features may include eye closing, wrinkled eyes, and a furrowed forehead. The pain cry has a shrill pitch and demands an immediate response.

External Pain. Similar to the cry of internal pain. The infant may start screaming suddenly without apparent reason. The infant also may have just awakened from a sound sleep.

Fever/illness. These cries tend to be of lower pitch and intensity. They have a whining, nasal quality and are prolonged in nature. An illness cry may elicit a more sympathetic response from the caregiver as opposed to the *red alert* response to the pain cry.

Anger. The angry cry has a vibrato quality of a sustained and lower pitch. You may hear hoarse sounds throughout the cry due to the turbulence of excess air being forced through the vocal cords. The lips and the mouth may be tightly clenched or pursed as compared with the open-mouth cry of the child in pain. You may see a snarled expression with arching of the back. The infant also may turn his or her head and push away. Possible reasons for an anger cry include being in an uncomfortable position, being dressed or undressed, or losing a pacifier.

Boredom. This cry has a whiny, low-pitched, moaning quality that does not necessarily set off an alarm to caregivers. You may hear occasional pauses as the infant expects the caregiver to come and give attention. This typically signals that the infant needs a change of activity, position, or type of interaction. This cry may sound fake and serve as a means of gaining the parent's attention.

Tension release from overstimulation. The infant's cry is prolonged and hard. The baby is generally unresponsive to efforts to comfort, such as nursing, rocking, or cuddling. This may be described as a letting-off-steam cry that generally is seen after a long over-stimulating day, particularly in the evening.

Fatigue. A tired infant's cry may start off slowly and proceed to one that is longer and has a notable vibrato quality. The eyes may be swollen slightly; the infant may rub the eyes.

Responses to Crying

Jones (1992) reported that some maternal conditions in pregnancy might contribute to an infant's high-pitched cry, including poor nutrition or toxemia. She further reported that this cry could reach seven to eight hundred cycles per second as opposed to a more typical cry of three to four hundred cycles per second. Children with other conditions such as prematurity, being small for the gestational age, or retardation may also contribute to a more irritating cry than that of typical children. Jones (1992) also reports that there is a higher incidence of abuse in these populations. It has been clinically observed that some neurologically involved infants have a different quality and pitch to their cries. Many parents and professionals report extreme difficulty in identifying a change in cry. This can make providing care, treatment, and interaction extremely frustrating. Parents, caregivers, and professionals should work together to identify cries and provide an appropriate response.

When determining your response to crying, it is important to consider

- the type of cry
- when the child last slept or was fed
- whether the child has symptoms of an illness or is teething
- the caregiver's sensitivity to crying
- any social factors that may cause stress for the child
- the preferences of the family
- the sensory environment
- the time of day

Crying and Massage

Massage is an interactive process between child and adult. If the child cries during the massage, the adult should respond by *modifying or stopping* the procedure.

Modifications may include changing the location, speed, pressure, or direction of the strokes. The adult may discontinue the massage and wait for another time, or briefly stop to change positions or allow the child to accommodate to the input already given. The child simply may need to be held, fed, or have the diaper changed. Continuing the massage through persistent crying is unlikely to be of therapeutic value and may have a negative impact on future massage interactions.

Although it is *not* recommended that massage begin while the child is crying, there are a few exceptions to the rule. If the crying continues although the child's physical needs have been met, gentle stroking may help alleviate the infant's discomfort. For example, caregivers instinctively stroke children's heads or backs to help calm them. Several parents have reported that after unsuccessfully trying everything else, they massaged their crying infant's stomach. The baby then produced a bowel movement or gas, which seemed to provide relief. Stroking can be combined with swaddling, gentle rocking, patting, or cuddling with the caregiver.

If the child is predominantly in the crying state when awake, the massage may have to be introduced despite the crying. The massage should be brief, with the goal of bringing the child to a more organized state. It is very important that the parents see some tangible sign of success. This may include a decrease in the intensity of the cry, muscular relaxation, or improved alertness/interaction.

Early massage experiences should be positive for both infant and caregiver. One public health nurse reported that she found it difficult to get mothers to continue with massage if their infants cried during the first experience. This may mean limiting the time and number of body parts covered, in the first few sessions based on the child's responses.

Crying is a challenging aspect of parenting. A parent's feeling of success or failure in consoling their child has significant implications for their parental confidence (Blackburn, 1989). A massage program can help parents and caregivers identify positions and strokes that aid in the child's organization and pleasure. In the long term, this will help promote consistent consolation and will boost parents' confidence in their handling and parenting skills.

Effects of Massage on State-Related Behaviors

Many parents and professionals find that consistent massage helps children modulate their sleep and wake states. Children who generally have irregular sleep cycles seem to sleep for longer periods of time and on a more consistent schedule.

Massage also appears to have a positive effect on state-related behaviors. Some infants and children appear to be more visually or auditorially alert during and/or after the massage. Many children increase their attempts to engage with the caregiver during the massage sessions, through vocalization, gestural communication, and socialization.

These subjective reports are supported by objective research findings (see Chapter 8). It is important to have a working knowledge of the infant's states and behaviors and to provide intervention according to the child's clues.

Summary

Massage is a useful tool to assist infants in state-related organization. Other sensory modalities such as vestibular, proprioceptive, visual, and auditory inputs also may be provided to achieve the desired response. It is critical to have a working knowledge of infant state and types of crying to provide the best sensory intervention for regulation.

To learn more about infant states and state-related behaviors, see Resources at the end of the text.

Chapter 5

The Autonomic Nervous System and Massage

Overview

The tactile system is primal to our well-being and ability to thrive (Montague, 1986), and it has a widespread effect on a child's general organizational ability, muscle tone, and behavior. By controlling pressure, temperature, direction, and speed of tactile input, one can help modulate behavioral state, physiological status, and tone. This offers interventionists and parents a powerful tool when working with a child with a neurological impairment. Massage also may enhance the functional performance of the child with an intact nervous system. Fritz (1995) said the basic premise of massage, with focus on the autonomic nervous system (ANS), is to provide for a balance of mind and body, allowing for efficient self-regulation. In addition to these benefits, there are marked improvements in adaptive behavior as a result of massage.

This chapter presents an overview of the ANS as it relates to the benefits of massage. For specific anatomical and physiological information, explore the various neurophysiological references in the bibliography.

Functional Anatomy

Two main divisions make up the ANS—the *parasympathetic* and the *sympathetic*. The divisions differ on an anatomical and functional level (Brodal, 1998). Their actions are often antagonistic; where one system dominates, the other reduces. However, there is increasing evidence supporting the concept that the two serve in a cooperative manner. The traditional model, describing the precise divisions of the ANS, is too simplistic. For the purposes of this chapter, the two divisions will be *generally* delineated according to functions, knowing that dynamic balance occurs between the two systems in an ongoing basis. This balance occurs most often without cortical awareness.

The sympathetic system functions in stress situations where mobilization of bodily resources is required. Conversely, the parasympathetic system contributes to maintenance processes such as digestion. The ANS works in synchrony with the endocrine system to control body physiology and promote homeostasis (Zigmond, Bloom, Landis, Roberts, & Squire, 1999). Cannon (1939) classically referred to the ANS as the "wisdom of the body."

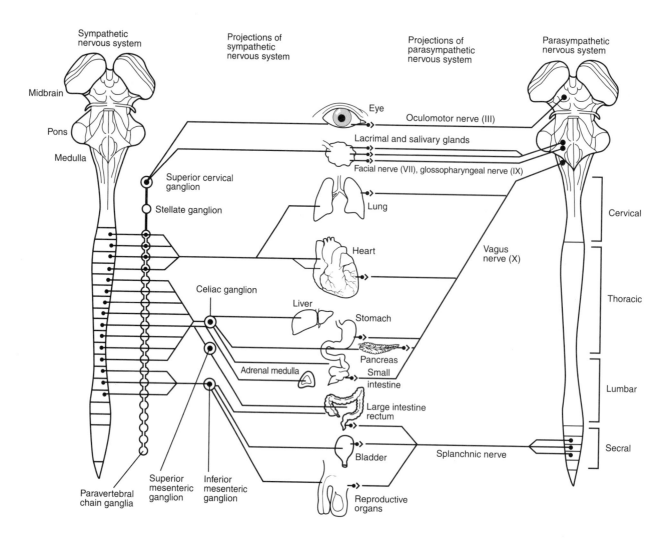

The ANS is based on a two-neuron chain with the preganglionic neuron located in the central nervous system and the postganglionic neuron located peripherally either in a ganglion or within the walls of a target organ. The ANS is divided according to the location of the preganglionic cell bodies.

The **parasympathetic** division of the ANS is classified as the *craniosacral* system, according to the location of the preganglionic cell bodies that arise from the cranial and sacral areas of the spinal cord. Conversely, the **sympathetic** division is classified as the thoracolumbar system, as its preganglionic cell bodies arise from the thoracic and lumbar areas of the spinal cord. The ganglia of the parasympathetic system are located close to the target organs, whereas the ganglia of the sympathetic system are located close to the central nervous system. Another distinction is the distribution of postganglionic fibers. Virtually all body parts receive sympathetic fibers, whereas the parasympathetic fibers are restricted primarily to the true visceral organs.

As a general rule, the **sympathetic division** is more *diffusely* organized compared with the more *precise* parasympathetic system (Brodal, 1998). This is reflected by comparing the relation and number of preganglionic and postganglionics of both systems. For example, in the parasympathetic ciliary ganglion, there are two postganglioninc fibers leaving the ganglion for each preganglionic fiber reaching it, producing a 2:1 relationship. Comparatively, the sympathetic superior cervical ganglion has a relationship of 30:1 in a cat and 60 to 90:1 in a human. This ganglion contains more than 1 million neurons in a human. This represents the extensive wiring of the sympathetic nervous system. Clinically, this is significant in that pronounced sympathetic functioning is hard-wired within the nervous system.

The differences between the structure and function may be illustrated with the following comparison (Zigmond, et al., 1999).

	Sympathetic division	Parasympathetic division
Location of preganglionic fibers	Thoracolumbar cord	Cranial neuroaxis, sacral cord
Location of postganglionic fibers	Distant from target organ	Near or in target organ
Postganglionic transmitter	Norepinephrine	Acetylcholine
Length of preganglionic axon	Relatively short	Relatively long
Length of postganglionic axon	Relatively long	Relatively short
Divergence of preganglionic axonal projection	One to many	One to few
Innervates trunk and limbs in addition to viscera	Yes	No

The Parasympathetic Division

We call upon the parasympathetic nervous system (PSNS) when sleeping, eating, and relaxing. Ernest Gellhorn (1967), a pioneer in exploration of the ANS, refers to the PSNS as the *trophotropic* system, meaning "toward nutrition." Powely (1999) described the PSNS as the rest-and-digest part of the nervous system. Additionally, Fritz (1995) described this system as restorative in nature and associated with a relaxation response. This contrasts to the typical fight-or-flight description of the sympathetic nervous system (SNS). The parasympathetic system works to (Brodal, 1998; Fritz, 1995; Zigmond, et al., 1999)

- enhance the restitution of cellular processes,

- decrease activity level,

- increase blood flow to the gastrointestinal system,

- promote the gastrointestinal process required to digest and absorb nutrients effectively,

- facilitate excretion and elimination of waste products,

- induce relaxation, and

- focus attention.

One typical parasympathetic response is the generalized relaxation felt after soaking in a hot tub.

The Sympathetic Division

The primary action of the sympathetic nervous system (SNS) is to expend energy such as the fight-or-flight response (Fritz, 1995). The early work of Gellhorn (1967) refers to the SNS as the *ergotropic* system, meaning "toward work." Stated most simply, the SNS functions primarily in emergency or stress-related situations. However, stimulation (e.g., subtle changes in emotions, sensory conditions, stress) can cause fluctuation on the continuum of autonomic responses. Powley (1999) describes the sympathetic system as mobilizing the resources of the body when extraneous effort is required. This may be seen as having great feats of strength as a result of SNS stimulation.

The sympathetic division creates the conditions for maximal performance through cardiovascular adjustments such as

- acceleration of heart rate,

- increase in force of heartbeat, and

- rise in arterial pressure.

The SNS prepares the body for emergency activity by (Brodal, 1998; Farber, 1982; Fritz, 1995; Gellhorn, 1967; Guyton, 1981; Pansky, 1988; Zigmond, et al., 1999)

- elevating blood sugar,

- delaying fatigue,

- dilating the bronchi,

- dilating the pupils, and

- increasing motor capacity by directing blood flow to the skeletal muscles at the expense of visceral and cutaneous circulation.

An example of a sympathetic response may be the anxiety people feel when they hear a police siren behind their mildly speeding car.

Balance Within the Autonomic Nervous System

The individual with central nervous system damage often will present with imbalanced ANS responses. Anecdotal reports from some clinicians suggest a correlation with pathology if one division of the ANS dominates. McCormack (1991) refers to this as pronounced sympathetic tone. The individual should be able to adaptively shift from one division to the other as necessary. It is helpful to view the ANS as a continuum of function, with the sympathetic and parasympathetic divisions at the extremes. The ideal functioning of the ANS in individuals would entail the ability to adaptively shift from one division to the other independently. Many clients require sensory intervention to achieve a more normalized state.

The concept of the continuum of function is challenged in that in many situations, both systems must be present for adequate functioning. For example, the sympathetic system is required for rising to stand from sitting, to avoid a fall in blood pressure. Thus, the sympathetic system's presence is crucial in daily life. McCormack (1991) described the destructive potential of prolonged sympathetic tone and its relation to the harm cycle. He described the initiation of the drug cortisol, a stress-related hormone, as the primary activator of the harm cycle. McCormack described the potential for hampering the immune system's function over time. Fritz (1995) described long-term levels of cortisol as causing similar effects as those attributable to cortisone (fluid retention, high blood pressure, impaired healing of wounds, vertigo, nausea, and headaches). She goes on to describe the exhaustion phase, when the body wears down and is more vulnerable to cardiac, respiratory, or gastrointestinal problems.

ANS and Massage

Ideally, a child should function within the norm and still have the ability to adaptively shift from one parameter of the ANS to the other. This is important in preserving body homeostasis and in regulating behavioral responses. Many children with neuromotor or sensory impairment experience extreme hyperirritability and inconsolability, with a reduced ability to return to a calm state once they have lost behavioral control. This may be associated with extreme extensor posturing when neuromotor impairment is present. These children may be functioning predominantly on the *sympathetic* side of the ANS. They present with difficulty in adaptively shifting their behavior toward a more organized and regulated response. Massage may be used in this case to lower the child's state and provide consolation.

The converse is the extremely lethargic child who is minimally interactive with the environment. This child may be functioning predominantly on the extreme *parasympathetic* side of the ANS. The child has difficulty adaptively shifting his or her behavior toward more alert and focused behavior. Massage may be instrumental in helping this child move toward a more optimal level of arousal and adaptive autonomic functioning.

Tappan (1998) described the *relaxation response* as a function of the parasympathetic nervous system. Specific benefits of the relaxation response as cited by Robbins, Powers, and Burgess (1994) include

- decreased oxygen consumption and metabolic rate, thus less strain on the body's energy resources;

- increased intensity and frequency of alpha brain waves associated with deep relaxation;

- reduced blood lactates (blood substances associated with anxiety);

- significantly decreased blood pressure in hypertensive individuals;

- reduced heart rate and slower respiration;

- decreased muscle tension;

- increased blood flow to the arms and legs;

- decreased anxiety, fears, and phobias, and increased positive mental health; and

- improved quality of sleep.

Tappan (1998) described soothing back massage in particular as having the quality to nurture, sympathize, and promote deep relaxation. She suggested that the nerves that exit the posterior vertebrae are easily triggered by massage to the back.

Neurotransmitters

Neurotransmitters are referred to in this text from a functional standpoint. Postganglionic fibers of the SNS are generally referred to as *adrenergic,* meaning that they use adrenaline/norepinephrine as a transmitter. Postganglionic fibers of the PSNS are generally referred to as *cholinergic*—they use acetylcholine as a transmitter (Brodal, 1998). This may be clinically significant because it takes longer for norepinephrine to dissipate from the bloodstream; thus, a sympathetic state may prevail. Some exceptions to these categories would best be described in the texts cited. The expansive *wiring* of the SNS also contributes to general activation of the sympathetic responses. Clinically, this may be seen as the child who has exceeded his or her limits and has extreme difficulty in returning to a calm state.

Involuntary Control

The ANS does not distinguish between real and apparent stress (Farber, 1982). For instance, the sympathetic portion of the nervous system may activate even if the danger is perceived but not real. Most autonomic responses take place without conscious control or awareness. However, techniques such as biofeedback and relaxation therapy have been used therapeutically to assist individuals in modulating autonomic responses.

It is important to be aware of the effects of stress on children and how their functional performance may be disrupted. Therapy procedures or treatment environments that may not seem stressful to the clinician may cause significant stress to the child and thus produce a sympathetic nervous system response.

Such procedures may include

- therapeutic casting of body parts

- changing the child's position

- changing the staff members who interact with the child

- range-of-motion procedures

- changing the sensory modality used or introducing a new therapy technique

- change of room temperature

- change in sensory stimulation of the room (i.e., more noise or bright lights)

Functions of the Parasympathetic and Sympathetic Systems

This chart is a synopsis of general functions of the parasympathetic and sympathetic nervous systems. Use it to determine the level of function of the child's autonomic nervous system. The information also can help you interpret the child's response to your tactile input before, during, and after the intervention (Barr & Kiernan, 1983; Brodal, 1998; Farber, 1982; Fritz, 1995; Guyton, 1981; Holmes & Lindsley, 1984; Kandell, Schwartz, & Jessel, 1991; Littel, 1990; Pansky, 1988).

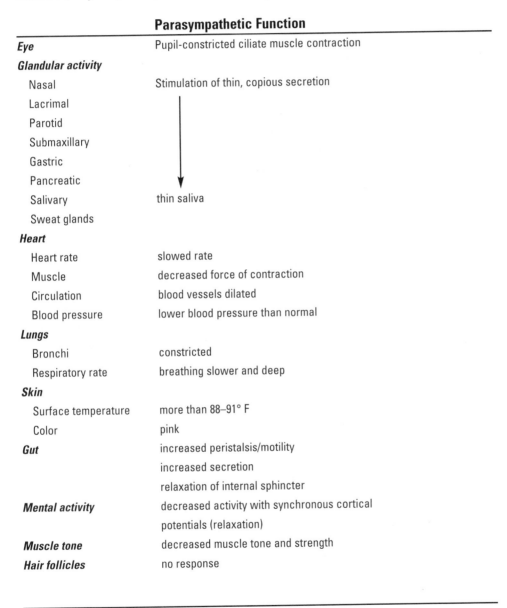

Parasympathetic Function	
Eye	Pupil-constricted ciliate muscle contraction
Glandular activity	
Nasal	Stimulation of thin, copious secretion
Lacrimal	
Parotid	
Submaxillary	
Gastric	
Pancreatic	
Salivary	thin saliva
Sweat glands	
Heart	
Heart rate	slowed rate
Muscle	decreased force of contraction
Circulation	blood vessels dilated
Blood pressure	lower blood pressure than normal
Lungs	
Bronchi	constricted
Respiratory rate	breathing slower and deep
Skin	
Surface temperature	more than 88–91° F
Color	pink
Gut	increased peristalsis/motility
	increased secretion
	relaxation of internal sphincter
Mental activity	decreased activity with synchronous cortical potentials (relaxation)
Muscle tone	decreased muscle tone and strength
Hair follicles	no response

Sympathetic Function

Eye	pupil dilated
	ciliary muscle slightly relaxed
Glandular activity	vasoconstriction and slight secretion
Nasal	
Lacrimal	
Parotid	
Submaxillary	
Gastric	
Pancreatic	
Salivary	dry mouth and thick saliva
Sweat glands	copious sweating
Heart	
Heart	increased rate and stroke volume
	dilation of the coronary arteries
Muscle	increased force of contraction
Circulation	vessels constricted
Blood pressure	increased blood pressure
Lungs	
Bronchi	vasodilated
Respiratory rate	breathing fast and shallow
Skin	
Surface temperature	less than 88–91° F when room is 79–81° F
Color	pale
Gut	decreased peristalsis/motility
	closure of the internal sphincter
	potential constipation
Mental activity	increased activity, synchronous cortical
	potentials, excitation or stress
Muscle tone	increased tone and strength
Hair follicles	excitation with hair standing on end, goose pimples

Measurement Criteria

The following are tangible indicators of ANS function.

Eyes	observe pupillary dilation/constriction observe visual gaze and tracking
Glands	observe the nasal and oral cavity for quality of secretion
Heart	monitor heart rate observe skin coloration
Lungs	monitor respiratory rate observe chest expansion during breathing monitor oxygen saturation
Skin	observe skin coloration measure skin temperature—stress dots are small dots that may be placed on the skin to determine skin temperature and associated stress
Gut	palpate abdomen inquire about frequency of elimination
Mental activity	observe child's orientation to environment, ability to focus
Muscle tone	use clinical measure of muscle tone

Range of Norms for Vital Signs

Consult your physician for a range of acceptable norms for the child. The medical condition and developmental stage vary for each child.

Altering Touch

A touch is characterized by a combination of qualities. Each quality can be adjusted to create massage strokes that please the child and help organize his or her adaptive responses. Changes in *pressure, direction, speed* or *frequency, temperature,* and *duration* influence the child's autonomic response.

The tactile system is made up of the *epicritic* system and the *protocritic* system. The protocritic system, previously called the protopathic system, develops first, followed by the fine discriminative properties of the epicritic system. These terms are used in this section to describe alteration in tactile input. Interaction between these systems occurs to balance the tactile response.

A variety of factors influence the dynamic balance of the two systems. These may include (but are not limited to)

- stress (physiological, somatic, behavioral, environmental)

- prior experience with touch (abuse, neglect, loving environment)

- integration of the current sensory system

- nutritional status

- bonding and attachment with the caregiver

- postural control

Pressure

Ryder (1988) describes deep-pressure touch as "a mechanical deformation of skin accompanied by underlying stimulation to the connective tissues and periosteum." Deep-pressure touch may be used to promote a parasympathetic nervous system response. McCormack (1991) described this pressure as between 5–10 milligrams of weight.

Umphred (1985) identifies the areas most sensitive to deep-pressure touch as the

- abdomen,

- perioral area,

- palms,

- soles of the feet, and

- paravertebral area.

Royeen and Lane (1991) described the role of the dorsal column medial lemniscal system and its balance between the anterolateral system. They suggested that deep pressure may impact modulation of arousal and have a calming effect. Deep-touch pressure and proprioception have been noted to have these properties. These sensations, in addition to vibration and touch pressure, are transmitted via the dorsal column. Conversely, the anterolateral system transmits information to mediate pain, crude touch, and temperature. Peele (1977) theorized that the dorsal column input may inhibit transmission in the anterolateral pathways, and the thalamus may be the site for this inhibition. This may account for the clinical implications of success in the use of deep-touch pressure to decrease pain and reduce tactile defensiveness. Additionally, anterolateral projections to the limbic and reticular systems, and the hypothalamus may account for respective changes in emotional tone, arousal, and autonomic regulation.

These areas have been empirically noted by Farber (1982) and Drehobl and Fuhr (1991) to elicit a parasympathetic relaxation response. Adults often use pressure in these areas to provide relief from stress by gripping their hands tightly, clasping their hands, and holding their hands around their mouth. People unconsciously provide their nervous system with tactile input to elicit calming. Children often react in the same way by biting, hand wringing, hand biting, or excessive contact of toys to the mouth. Massage may help provide this deep-touch pressure, eliciting a parasympathetic response and calming.

The palm of the hand makes a good massage tool because it provides even pressure. Try this comparison: place your relaxed palm on your face. Now place just your fingertips on your face. Compare the stimuli; note the even input provided by the palm.

A smaller surface area produces a more concentrated response. The child with hypersensitivity will be acutely aware of multiple tactile inputs; thus, it is important to assure direct and even pressure.

Strokes involving deep pressure will most likely produce the calming effect desired for a child with hypersensitivity.

Some deep-pressure strokes include

- Indian Milking,
- Paddle Wheel,
- Pressure on the Abdomen,
- Pressure on Soles of Feet,

- Back and Forth,
- Swooping,
- Heart, and
- Criss-Cross.

By contrast, light-touch pressure is a *protocritic stimulus,* as it tends to promote a facilatory response or alert the central nervous system. Light touch may be used therapeutically for increasing arousal in the minimally interactive child, but it may be overwhelming or disorganizing for the hypersentive child or child with high tone. Be sure to have a clear assessment of the child's sensory functioning and muscle tone before proceeding with light-touch pressure.

Because light touch is a powerful stimulus, it must be used cautiously when combined with other therapeutic modalities. Light touch may elicit aversive responses in anyone whose nervous system is not yet prepared to accommodate it. At first, use only firm-pressure strokes. Subsequently, evaluate the child's response when adding strokes that use light or varied touch pressures.

The neonate functions primarily on the protocritic level of touch because more mature sensations have not developed yet. Therefore, neonates may be stimulated more easily by massage strokes. It is important to note that a neonate's tolerance for touch intervention is lower than that of an adult, due to the densely packed sensory receptors per square inch of skin. Be aware of the infant's response to touch and adjust intervention accordingly. Some light-touch strokes include Swedish milking (second phase) and combing.

Direction

According to Gellhorn (1967), the direction of the stroking has important implications for the function of the autonomic nervous system. The work of Margaret Rood also incorporated principles of directional touch in her "fast brushing and slow stroking" (Farber, 1982). This work has been expanded via clinical observation and research.

Longworth (1982) described the use of repetetive slow stroking down the back, provided over a time period of 6 minutes, to lower autonomic arousal. If this stimulation occurred over the long term, decreased psycho-emotional and somatic arousal were noted. Simply stated, smooth directional pressure assists in calming. The strokes presented in this text are a combination of Swedish strokes (moving distally to proximally) and Indian strokes (moving proximally to distally).

Strokes moving in a slow, rhythmical manner with the direction of hair growth produce a calming or inhibitory response. This may serve to calm children with hypersensitivity and reduce stiffness in the child with hypertonicity. These strokes include

- Indian Milking,
- Stroking from shoulders to hands,

- Stroking from shoulders (over the trunk and legs) to feet, and
- Swooping.

These generalizations should be validated by clinical observation of the child being treated. Further, controlled research is needed to confirm these clinical observations.

Conversely, the child with hypotonicity or lethargy may benefit from strokes against the hair growth, which tend to facilitate increased proximal activation of muscles and promote arousal. The interventionist needs to evaluate individual responses to ensure that they are not aversive. However, the best determination is to continually evaluate the child's adaptive response to the sensory input, with specific goals to address the therapeutic needs. Examples of strokes-against-the-hair pattern include Swedish milking (first phase) and stroking the top of the foot.

The child with hair whorls is an exception to this principle. Massage over the site of hair whorls may be disorganizing to the child.

Speed/Frequency

The speed and frequency of stroking may be altered to produce a desired effect. Each child's response to stroking should be assessed individually and altered, as necessary.

Brisk or arrhythmical stroking done at a high speed and frequency tends to facilitate tone (Drehobl & Fuhr, 1991). A brisk, arrhythmical quality can be incorporated into the following strokes:

- Rolling,
- Swedish Milking, and
- Combing.

Slow, rhythmical stroking tends to relax the muscles of a child with hypertonicity, and facilitate overall relaxation. Some even, rhythmical strokes are

- Indian Milking,
- Swooping, and
- Back and forth.

Temperature

The temperature of the interventionist's hands is critical in producing a response to massage. Cold hands or a cool room may elicit a sympathetic nervous system response and promote behaviors such as increased tone and irritability, negating the purpose of the massage. Before starting the massage, warm your hands in warm water or in front of a hand dryer or heater, or use biofeedback. You also can use a microwaveable neck warmer to warm your hands.

The environment should be warm enough to preserve the child's body temperature. This may be accomplished by:

- draping body parts not involved in the massage,

- keeping a piece of clothing on the child,

- warming blankets or towels in a dryer, and

- increasing the room temperature.

Duration of Stimulus

Rebound (overcompensation) is a possibility when using the sensation of touch to modulate autonomic response. Als, Lester, and Tronick (1982) advocated observation before, during, and after an intervention.

Be sure to monitor the child's baseline status, behavior during tactile intervention, and subsequent effect of massage. "If one uses too many calming techniques on a patient, his body processes may speed up in an attempt to restore homeostasis" (Gellhorn, 1967). This is particularly important for the medically fragile child or the premature infant. The interventionist should take great care to elicit greater organization and adaptive responses without eliciting a stress response.

As with any therapy technique, the interventionist should introduce handling in an organized and sequential manner, carefully observing the child's responses. To assure carrythrough and have the child associate touch with pleasure, it is important that initial massage intervention be positive.

Introduce massage to one body part per session. This gives the child time to process the input, and the caregivers an opportunity to practice. However, this needs to be assessed individually with each child. If your therapy goal includes enhancement of the total body scheme, a full-body massage would be appropriate.

Implications for Massage

The ANS holds important implications for the use of massage. Variation in pressure, direction, temperature, and speed of touch may be used to facilitate developmentally appropriate adaptive responses. It is important to have a thorough understanding of the child's sensory and motor needs before initiating massage. Pay close attention to the child's behavior and physical cues of over- or understimulation. Document your findings to determine progress toward specific goals.

Chapter 6

Signs and Symptoms of Overstimulation

Adaptive Responses

A goal of massage for infants and children is to provide a *natural,* yet *controlled,* sensory experience that enables the child to produce an adaptive response. The words *natural* and *controlled* are very important in describing the method in which we approach massage for children. Massage is a natural extension of caring touch. However, it is critical that we be aware of, control, and monitor the aspects of touch. Tactile input is a powerful sensory tool influencing many body systems, behavior, and self-organization. Careful attention is paid to the child's response to the input before, during, and after massage. The qualities of the touch are altered accordingly or the touch may be discontinued.

Farber (1982) defined *adaptive response* as behavior that is more advanced, organized, flexible, or productive in nature, resulting from the application of a sensory intervention. An adaptive response should be developmentally appropriate. Fisher, Murray, and Bundy (1991) stated that the broader term *adaptive behavior* implies that an individual freely chooses between several effective strategies. They further elaborated that adaptive behaviors are organized and planned. They include cognitive, motor, and postural skills.

Some potential adaptive responses and behaviors that may be facilitated through the massage process are

- elongation of soft tissues to prepare the child for more efficient movement

- deeper respiration

- improved circulation of the extremities

- decreased sensory defensiveness

- enhanced social interaction with the caregiver

- improved gastrointestinal function

- increased quality or quantity of vocalization/communication

- improved visual orientation with the caregiver

- more efficient feeding

- more sustained attention

- improved ability to console or regulate behavior

The literature presented in this chapter will help assess the child's communication of pleasure or distress. This information can be used as a guideline to gauge the appropriateness and effectiveness of the massage.

Guidelines for the Preterm Infant

Advanced Skills

A common goal of gentle touch in the nursery is to facilitate parent-infant contact and enhance the development of the parent-infant relationship. However, because of the medical fragility of preterm infants, professionals supporting them and their parents in the Neonatal Intensive Care Unit (NICU) need to have advanced training, extensive knowledge, and current skills. The person offering massage to preterm infants (preferably the parent) must be aware of potential adverse physiological effects such as apnea, bradycardia, excessive expenditure of energy, and decreased oxygen saturation levels. Vandenberg (1993) stated that sick neonates must be able to maintain autonomic nervous system balance before they are able to modulate sensory input. Fragile infants who are not physiologically stable can be easily overwhelmed by any stimuli, including tactile. VandenBerg also described some of the competencies needed for developmental specialists to optimally support and communicate the behavioral needs of the infant.

One type of advanced training that may be obtained is the use of the *neurobehavioral approach*. Als and Gilkerson (1997) describe this as a developmentally supportive, relationship-based approach to newborn intensive care with the goal of enhancing the strengths of the family and infant. Referred to as the Newborn Individualized Developmental Care and Assessment Program (NIDCAP®) (Als, 1986), it provides detailed behavioral observations and individualized recommendations for caregiving based on the infant's level of functioning and inferred goals. It is a supportive and collaborative process with the infant, parent, and professional.

The NIDCAP was the foundation for the development of the *Infant Behavioral Assessment* (Hedlund & Tatarka, 1988) and the *Neurobehavioral Curriculum for Early Intervention* (Hedlund, 1996). The assessment and curriculum are used with infants from birth through 6 months of developmental age, with very low birthweight or at risk for poor, long-term neuro-developmental outcome. One goal of this approach is to provide support for early interventionists to read and interpret the infant's behavioral story (Als, 1997). The infant's behavior offers continual information about his or her ability to interact with caregivers and the environment. This behavioral story can relay information about the infant's goals, strategies they use to accomplish goals, effectiveness of the strategies, and supports necessary to enhance the infant's development and neurobehavioral organization. Information about these professional trainings is listed in the Resources on page 173.

Research

Research with preterm infants has shown variable outcomes depending upon the type of tactile intervention offered and the characteristics of the infants, including physiological stability, maturity, and health status. In most of the studies, someone other than the parent provided the touch intervention. Also, most treatment took place in the NICU (except Rice, 1979) and followed a prescribed routine rather than being responsive to the infant's cues. Several early studies of massage with physiologically stable, preterm infants reported

- increased weight gain (Field, Scafidi, & Schanberg, 1987; Field, et al.,1986; Rausch, 1981; Rice, 1979; White & Labarba, 1976)

- improved socialization (Kramer, Chamorro, Green, & Knudtson,1975; Rice, 1979)

- improved ability to achieve a quiet alert state (White-Traut & Pate, 1987)

- enhanced development (Field, Scafidi, & Schanberg, 1987; Field et al., 1986)

- more quiet sleep (Strong, 1989)

Other studies have reported that gentle human touch did not seem to harm the infants (Harrison, Olivet, Cunningham, Bodin, & Hicks, 1996; Jay, 1982; White-Traut & Tubeszewski, 1986). Further research is presented in Chapter 8.

Pediatric massage and gentle touch pressure as described in this book differ from the tactile intervention given in research studies in that it is interactive and dependent upon the infant's behavioral cues and physiological response.

Definitions of Types of Tactile Input

Difficulty in interpreting the results from research and clinical observations may arise due to variability in defining the type of the tactile intervention employed. Modrcin-McCarthy, Harris, and Marlar (1997) discussed the benefits and risks of various types of comforting touch techniques, including

- **massage** (gentle rubbing of a portion of the infant's body)

- **stroking** (rhythmic, repetitive, movement of the palm or fingers over a portion of the body)

- **tactile/kinesthetic input** (combination of stroking or massage with passive flexion/extension movements)

- **gentle human touch** (continuous touch with gentle hand placement on the infant's body)

- **kangaroo care** (skin-to-skin contact with the infant placed inside the parent's shirt)

They examined numerous research studies involving preterm infants to analyze the potential stimulatory levels of each of these types of touch techniques. Massage, stroking, and tactile/kinesthetic input were found to be the most potentially stimulating. Kangaroo care was considered to have a moderate or low potential stimulatory level while gentle human touch was determined to have a low level. Therefore, gentle human touch may be more appropriate for smaller, more fragile, and less mature infants than massage, stroking, or tactile/kinesthetic touch. They concluded that the benefits and negative effects of touch are related to the individual characteristics of the preterm infant and the type of touch used.

Responding to Cues

Modrcin-McCarthy, Harris, and Marlar (1997) suggested that vital signs should be closely monitored and the infant should be observed for signs of overstimulation. White-Traut and Goldman (1988) suggested that if an infant exhibits negative behavioral cues (i.e., fussing, crying, increased hypertonicity or motor activity, color changes, or vomiting) or unacceptable autonomic responses (unacceptable vital sign changes) during massage to a particular area, then that body part should not be massaged. The massage should be discontinued if the negative cues persist for more than a minute. Always use this conservative approach of constant monitoring.

A 1985 study by Oehler examined talking, touching, and talking combined with touching, with preterm infants who were divided into three groups: well, sick, and moderately ill. The well infants showed more smiling and hand-to-mouth activity during the three types of stimulus than the moderately ill or sick infants. The sick infants displayed the greatest avoidance during the combination of talking and touching. Oehler suggested that sick infant's parents provide only one type of stimulation at a time. She concluded that for sick infants, talking might be safer and more likely to produce alertness than touching.

These guidelines can be used to provide interventionists, caregivers, and parents with concrete observations of the infant's behavioral response throughout the massage or touch process.

Stress Signals

In order to provide organizing tactile input, the facilitator must

- constantly monitor the child's physiological and behavioral cues, and
- modify or stop the input based on the child's responses.

The caregiver should monitor the infant's behavior before, during, and after the intervention. In order for massage to be *effective and safe* it is *critical* that the infant's signs of self-regulation and potential overstimulation be monitored. As described in Als, et al. (1982), the signs and symptoms of overstimulation can be observed on three different levels of stress signals: autonomic and visceral, motoric, and state-related.

Autonomic and Visceral Stress Signals

Observe breathing and color. Stress signals may include

- seizure activity
- respiratory irregularities
- color changes
- spitting up

- hicupping
- yawning
- startling
- tremoring

Vital signs are indicators of physiological stability. Monitors should be scanned for information about heart and respiratory rates, oxygen saturation, or blood pressure as concrete measures of physiological status.

Motoric Stress Signals

Be aware of extremity, trunk, and facial behaviors. Motoric stress signals may include

- flaccidity of trunk and extremities;

- hyperextension of extremities, trunk, or tongue;

- frantic activity, squirming, or twitching;

- legs or feet extending toward a surface as if attempting to stabilize (bracing postures);

- the high guard arm position;

- grimacing; and

- extreme flexion postures.

State-Related Stress Signals

Observe clusters of behaviors (including eye opening and eye movements, facial expressions, postural tone, gross body movements, and respiration) to determine the infant's level of consciousness. State-related stress signals may include

- irritability

- fussing or crying

- eye floating, averting, or staring

- sleeplessness

- disorganization of infant states (Refer to Chapter 4 for more information.)

It is important to re-emphasize the need to modify or discontinue the massage if stress signals are observed. These signals may be the infant's means of self-protection or avoidance of environmental stressors as well as ways to communicate overstimulation. Recognition of early signs of stress must be identified to optimize an infant's response to massage. *Overstimulation may prove unsafe for medically fragile or premature infants.*

Listening to Infants

Engagement and Disengagement

The *Nursing Child Assessment Satellite Training Learning Resource Manual* (NCAST) (Barnard, 1989) described ways to respond to infants' verbal and nonverbal communication. Refer to the NCAST programs and materials for in-depth information about infant communication. (See the NCAST listing in Resources.) Ericks (1989) used the terms *engagement* and *disengagement* to represent the infant's readiness for interaction. This is highly useful in determining your interaction and massage intervention with an infant.

Engagement

Infants offer subtle and strong signals of engagement that indicate that they are ready for interaction. Look for these verbal and nonverbal cues as the infant's communication before you begin the massage.

Subtle engagement cues are the infant's initial readiness signs that may include

- facial alerting signs—eyes may widen, eyebrows raise, and face brighten;
- head-lifting and eyes turning toward you; and
- hands open with the fingers relaxed and slightly flexed.

A quieting of movement in the arms or legs may indicate anticipation. (Quieting of movement also may be a subtle disengagement cue.)

Potent engagement cues are strong signs that the infant is ready for interaction. They may include

- verbal readiness cues—giggling, babbling, talking, or making feeding sounds;
- smiling; and
- sustained eye-to-eye contact or looking at your face.

Movements of the extremities generally will be smooth. The infant may turn the head toward you or reach toward you to indicate readiness.

Disengagement

Infants also offer subtle and strong cues of disengagement, which indicate a need for a break in the interaction. Respect this communication! If you observe the following signals during a massage, modify your technique or stop.

Subtle disengagement cues are the first signals that the infant needs a break in the interaction. They may include

- whimpering, yawning, or hicupping;
- an increase in sucking noises;
- facial grimacing, frowning, or pouting;
- head lowering and eyes closing;
- eyes turning away from you, closing tightly, or blinking rapidly;
- shoulders elevating;
- arms held close to the stomach while the hands move over the trunk as if searching;
- increased kicking, foot movement, or diffuse body movement; and
- legs straightening tightly or the arms straightening alongside the body. (Conversely, a quieting or movement of the arms and legs also could be a subtle disengagement cue.)

You also may notice subtle fine-motor disengagement cues such as

- bringing a hand to an ear, the stomach, the back of the neck, or the mouth;
- joining the hands together over the stomach while engaging in finger manipulation;
- grasping the body, clothing, or both forearms; and
- rotating the wrist rapidly.

Potent disengagement cues are strong or secondary signs that an infant needs a break in the interaction. Strong verbal cues can include

- crying, whining, fussing
- choking or vomiting

Strong motoric disengagement cues can include

- back arching;
- turning the head and gazing away;
- pulling away;
- attempts at pushing you away or shaking the head *no*; and
- rolling, crawling, or walking away.

Withdrawing from an alert state to a sleep state is another potent disengagement cue.

These cues can help you determine the infant's readiness for massage as well as the infant's response to the intervention. Let the infant give you active cues for the initiation of strokes, communication of pleasure, and information about when to end the massage. For example, you can interpret subtle or potent cues of engagement, such as smiling or a mutual gaze, as your signal that the infant is ready to interact.

Subtle disengagement cues may be the initial signal that the infant's limits are approaching. Let that be your cue to taper off the massage; end it by holding or gently interacting with the infant. Concluding a massage with the infant giving potent disengagement cues, such as crying or back arching, may be stressful for the family. Try to complete the massage *before* the infant gives strong negative cues so that the experience will be more positive for everybody.

The older, verbal child will be able to communicate responses to massage with statements such as

- "More!"
- "Rub my back!"
- "That feels nice."
- "Stop!"

Crying

Crying is a fundamental communication of stress or overstimulation that must be respected. The person providing the tactile intervention must analyze this response and modify the technique accordingly. See Chapter 4 for more information about crying.

Modifying the Massage Experience

Crying or other stress signals are clear indicators that you need to modify the massage experience. You may

- respond to the child's physiological needs such as hunger, thirst, or the need to be held. **Physiological needs always take precedence over the massage!**

- increase or decrease the pressure being used;

- reduce the speed of the stroke;

- change the location of the tactile input;

- use a different type of stroke such as a long sweeping stroke (milking) instead of a wringing motion;

- move the child to a more comfortable position;

- make sure the temperature of the room, support surface, and your hands are comfortable;

- use a bathmit or soft soap to provide massage while bathing;

- use an alternative calming technique, such as vestibular input (slow rocking), proprioceptive input (bouncing or deep pressure), or rhythmical music;

- decrease extraneous visual or auditory stimuli;

- offer gentle-touch pressure (placing a relaxed hand on the child's abdomen, head, or other body part);

- provide swaddling for neutral warmth;

- use an alternative medium for massage, such as the child's favorite blanket; and

- discontinue the massage until a later time.

Summary

In order for the touch experience to be most beneficial to the infant, the provider must be knowledgeable, choose an appropriate level or type of tactile input, monitor the infant's behavioral and physiological signs, and respond accordingly.

Chapter 7

Medical Considerations

Introduction

Tactile intervention is a powerful therapeutic tool for health care professionals, educators, and parents. The practitioner must know when massage is advised *and* when it may be potentially harmful. Proceed only with a thorough working knowledge of the child's medical history and any potential contraindications. **Consult the child's primary physician before initiating the massage program to determine possible risks and discuss goals. You also may need to contact specialists in complex medical situations.**

To have a safe, effective, and enjoyable experience, you should use a conservative approach in the use of massage for infants and children with special needs. The introduction of massage appears to have had a positive effect on the physical and emotional well-being of these children.

Nevertheless, massage could pose a risk to the health of children who have medical conditions. **This chapter is *not* intended to offer medical advice.** It *is* intended to give basic information about the use of tactile intervention in the presence of illness or medical disorders. It is hoped that this chapter will not frighten or discourage you from providing massage to children with special needs. Rather, this knowledge will facilitate appropriate clinical decision-making about the most beneficial use of touch.

You may never encounter some of the medical conditions described, but it is important to understand the rationale behind the contraindications they present. These general principles then may be applied to other disorders. Often, however, even when massage or stroking is contraindicated, a gentle placing of hands on the child may be comforting.

Many of the contraindications found in the literature are based on traditional knowledge and the practitioner's experience. Research and scientific evidence are only recently emerging. Therefore, different references vary in their recommendations regarding medical contraindications and indications for massage. The following definitions will be used in this book.

A *contraindication*, as used in this chapter, means the presence of a condition that makes massage potentially undesirable or harmful and is therefore inadvisable.

Indication is used to describe situations and conditions in which massage will not harm the child and may be beneficial or helpful.

The following definitions and questions may be helpful in determining appropriateness of massage:

1. Will the type of massage increase circulation?

   Circulatory massage is stroking or kneading of the muscles at medium to deep pressure, which moves blood and lymph through the tissues. Walton (1998, p. 110–111) defined this further as "medium or deep pressure includes any pressure that is greater than simple, resting-hand contact on the skin: it displaces muscle or fat tissue and puts mechanical pressure on the deeper vessels below. In light pressure, mechanical manipulation is limited to the structures of the skin." One needs to determine whether the child's system can handle increased blood flow through a specific area and/or the entire body.

2. What location on the body is the massage to be performed?

   A **local massage** is directly on the injured or diseased area, **regional massage** is around the area, and a **general massage** is anywhere on the body.

   There are many situations (e.g., fractures, burns, open wounds) in which massage is contraindicated at the site of the injury, condition, or disease, but may be used elsewhere on the body to promote relaxation and improve circulation to the healing area.

3. What is the stage of the illness or injury?

   Acute means relatively severe and short-term.

   Sub-acute means between acute and chronic and is usually of mild severity and duration.

   Chronic means persisting over a long duration.

   There are a number of conditions (e.g., scar tissue, psoriasis, inflammation due to arthritis) where local massage is contraindicated in the acute phase but may be helpful in the sub-acute or chronic phase. Also, although a full-body massage is not recommended during a severe asthma episode, it can be very helpful in teaching relaxation between episodes, which may help decrease the severity and length of future episodes.

4. What is the underlying cause of the condition?

   In some situations, the reason for the condition determines whether massage is appropriate, and if so, what type and location. For example, edema (swelling) due to heart, liver, or kidney conditions is a contraindication for general massage. If it is due to trauma, local massage is contraindicated. However, if the edema is due to inactivity or immobilization, massage may be indicated.

5. Is the child taking any medications?

   The person giving the massage needs to be aware of any medications that change sensation, arousal level, muscle tone, or cardiovascular, liver, or kidney function, and contact the child's physician prior to massage. Some types of medications that may be problematic in association with massage include anti-inflammatories, pain relievers, muscle relaxants, and blood thinners (anti-coagulants). Some types of massage can increase or decrease the effectiveness of various medications. Children may not be able to accurately perceive pain when taking analgesics, and therefore, may be unreliable in communicating their response to tactile input. If there is a concern about medication and the use of massage, the child's pediatrician should be contacted.

The following is a general summary of contraindications; however, the chart and discussion will further elaborate on this subject.

- Acute conditions requiring first aid or medical attention are contraindications for massage.

- Massage is contraindicated for systemic contagious or infectious conditions.

- Acute, unstable, or advanced conditions of the heart, kidney, or liver are contraindications for massage. Circulatory/respiratory conditions or failure also are contraindications for massage.

Although skin-to-skin contact is preferred, gloves may be used to prevent viral or bacterial infection between the massage giver and the child. (It should be noted that latex gloves may break down and be ineffective if oil is used.) Latex gloves may produce severe allergic reactions in some children and adults. Wash hands thoroughly before and after every massage to protect both the massage giver and the child.

The following are situations in which a full-body massage, including stroking that may increase circulation, is contraindicated. These are standard contraindications. However, there are conditions that recent research is addressing that are indicated with an asterisk. More information about these conditions can be located in the research chart in Chapter 8.

Acute Infections

If the child has an acute infection, the physician should be contacted and appropriate medical care prescribed before considering massage in a treatment program. Although massage is not recommended if the child has an acute infection, simply placing your relaxed hands over the child's forehead, back, or abdomen may be soothing.

Massage generally is contraindicated in the case of acute infection for several reasons.

- Massage could spread the infection to surrounding tissues.

- Children usually do not respond well to massage when they are ill. Their tolerance of touch, especially stroking, may be lower at this time.

- Interaction between the child and caregiver may be limited due to the child's lethargy or discomfort.

The list that follows provides some examples of acute infections and their symptoms/etiology. The definitions used in this chapter are a synthesis of information from the references listed under *Development/Medicine/Neurophysiology* unless otherwise credited.

Abnormal body temperature. Elevated temperature may indicate the presence of infection. Other obvious signs of infection, such as pulling on the ears, sore throat, or a skin lesion, may accompany a fever. If the child feels warm or feverish before the massage, take the child's body temperature as a precaution. Some practitioners recommend avoiding massage if the child's temperature is above 100.5° F. Fever occurs when the child's defense mechanism is impacted by various infectious and noninfectious processes (Nelson, Behrman, Kliegman, & Arvin, 1996). Contact the child's physician.

Influenza. The *flu* is a viral infection of the respiratory tract characterized by an abrupt onset of fever, chills, cough, headache, fatigue, nasal discharge, muscle aches, and occasional nausea. The child's physician may have specific recommendations to increase comfort. Additionally, a gentle hand placed on the forehead, back, or abdomen may comfort the child. When symptoms lessen and with physician approval, give a gentle massage to the chest, back, and face. This may help relieve congestion.

Pertussis. Recently there have been isolated outbreaks of pertussis or *whooping cough.* Some children with health or neurological problems have not been immunized against this disease. Pertussis is a very contagious acute infection of the respiratory tract. It usually is characterized initially by a slight fever, runny nose, sneezing, sore eyes, and a dry cough. In the second stage, the cough is characterized by a series of rapid, short coughs and a deep, high-pitched inspiration. Pertussis is a very serious and possibly fatal infection. Medical attention is imperative.

Severe respiratory infections or colds. Symptoms of respiratory infections may include fever, cough, and chest pain. Symptoms of a cold include runny nose, sore throat, fever, cough, and headache. Medical treatment is determined by the severity of the symptoms. In severe cases, massage is contraindicated. A gentle hand placement on the back, forehead, or abdomen may be comforting to the child with a less severe infection. The child's physician may feel that gentle massage to the face, chest, and back is appropriate to help relieve congestion.

Staph infections. Staph infections are a group of infections that are caused by staphylococci bacteria, which may cause skin or wound infections or serious internal disorders, including pneumonia and meningitis. Massage is contraindicated in the case of staph because it is highly contagious. Medical treatment is necessary.

Tuberculosis. Tuberculosis is a disease that is transmitted from person to person usually by airborne mucus droplets. Symptoms of primary pulmonary tuberculosis in children may be minimal, even when radiographic changes are moderate to severe. Infants are more likely to display signs and symptoms, including nonproductive cough and dyspnea. Fever, night sweats, weight loss, wheezing, and a decrease in activity may occur. Tuberculosis in children with HIV infection often is more severe. A positive tuberculin skin test, abnormal chest radiograph, and history of exposure is considered adequate proof of diagnosis (Nelson, 1996; Behrman, Kliegman, & Arvin, 1996). Anti-tuberculosis medication is given for a prolonged period and requires adherence to the regimen. Werner and Benjamin (1998) reported that massage is contraindicated for active tuberculosis, unless the client has physician's approval and has been on consistent medication for several weeks.

Cardiac and Circulatory Conditions

When using massage for the child with cardiac and circulatory conditions, the child's physician must provide approval to rule out any potential risk. The child's circulatory system may not be able to accommodate the increased volume of blood flow through the heart and accompanying vessels created by the pumping action of the long, firm strokes toward the heart.

Massage also could pose the risk of dislodging a clot and causing subsequent severe neurological or cardiac damage. In the case of recent heart surgery or cardiac instability, a gentle placement of your hands on the child's forehead, back, abdomen, or extremities may be comforting.

Not all cardiac conditions are contraindications for massage. However, it is *critical* that you consult the physician about the child's stability before proceeding with massage. An example might be in the case of a child with Down syndrome who has recovered from successful surgery for congenital cardiac anomalies. The heart may present no complication, and massage may be an appropriate part of a therapy or home program.

The following are examples of circulatory and cardiac conditions and their implications for massage.

Edema. Edema is the accumulation of fluid in the interstitial space and may be associated with inflammatory and circulatory causes (Werner & Benjamin, 1998). Consult the child's physician to determine the nature of the edema and the appropriateness of massage. The type, location, and cause of edema will determine whether massage is indicated. Massage is contraindicated for most edemas, especially if the edema is pitting.

To test for *pitting edema,* apply firm finger pressure to the skin over the edematous area. Pitting edema is present if an indentation remains after the finger has been removed. The fluid moves from the area where the pressure is applied to other tissue. The indentation usually takes several seconds to return to the level of the adjoining skin (Beck, 1994).

Generally, massage is indicated only if the edema results from subacute soft-tissue injury or temporary immobilization, which is caused by another condition that is not contraindicated.

Massage is contraindicated if the edema is due to (1) heart, liver, or kidney conditions, (2) infection, or (3) mechanical blockage anywhere in the circulatory system (Werner & Benjamin, 1998).

Hemophilia. This is a genetic disorder that affects blood clotting. It is characterized by hematomas, persistent bleeding, or hemorrhaging into the joints. This may be due to relatively minor trauma, but also may appear spontaneously (Nelson,

1996; Behrman, Kliegman, & Arvin, 1996). Massage is contraindicated, as it may cause further bruising or internal bleeding.

Hematoma. Hematoma is a localized collection of blood that is usually clotted in an organ, space, or tissue. It is caused by bleeding from a break in the wall of the blood vessel. Massage should not be given over the site of purple or blue bruises, and is contraindicated when there are internal injuries, avoiding further injury.

High blood pressure. Consult with the physician if the child has a history of elevated blood pressure or is currently receiving medication for hypertension. Gentle hand placements as previously described may be appropriate, as they do not increase the blood flow.

Very low blood pressure. Conversely, very low blood pressure also may be a contraindication for massage due to the possibility of fainting. Individuals with very low blood pressure should rise slowly from a seated or lying position after massage (Tappan, 1998).

Skin Disorders

The following skin conditions may be contraindications for massage. Some of the conditions listed apply only to isolated areas; other parts of the body may be safely massaged. Massage should not be given in the case of a contagious skin disease, as the disease could be exacerbated. Interventionists also should be aware of the potential health risk to them and use precautions (e.g., gloves) as necessary.

Skin allergies. Consult the child's physician before using oil. The primary caregiver also will know whether the child has had any previous reactions to oils or lotions. Lubrication may further irritate the affected area and result in infection. To determine sensitivity, a simple skin-patch test should be performed. (Refer to Chapter 10 for information about skin-patch testing.)

Localized skin disorders. In localized skin conditions, only the affected area is of concern and needs to be avoided during massage. Localized skin disorders include but are not limited to

- acne/pimples, blisters, boils, broken vessels, bruises, scratches, skin tags, warts.

- burns*. After open wounds have healed and the risk of infection is eliminated, consult the child's physician about the use of massage to keep skin supple and in an optimal state of nutrition.

- open wounds or sores. Do not massage over the site of an open wound. This may spread infection to the surrounding tissues and potentially to you.

- skin lesions or growths that continue to grow or bleed, lumps, moles, scaly patches, and tumors. A physician should examine these.

Basal cell carcinoma, the most common form of skin cancer, is very rare in children. Since it seldom metastasizes, massage that avoids the cancerous area may be appropriate with physician approval. Massage is contraindicated in the case of malignant melanoma. Some resources believe that the increase in circulation could potentially metastasize the cancer. A gentle placement of your relaxed hands on unaffected areas may be comforting. The hand placement does not increase circulation.

Massaging the open lesions of skin disorders could precipitate an infection. The following conditions could be aggravated by the lubricant used or by the massage itself. In some situations, it may be possible to massage unaffected areas.

Dermatitis*. Dermatitis is an inflammation of the skin. Causes include eczema, psoriasis, and seborrhea. The condition of the skin and cause of the inflammation determine whether massage is appropriate. For example, massage may be helpful for dry, flaky eczema but would be contraindicated if the inflammation has lesions or could spread.

Hypersensitive skin. Massage is contraindicated if the child has hypersensitive skin that may be further aggravated. Massage may be given without oil or lotion if it is the lubrication that causes the problem. Massage also may be given through clothes, pajamas, or a blanket.

Contagious skin disorders. In many contagious skin conditions, massage poses the risk of further aggravating the tissues and should be avoided. There also is the risk of transfer of the condition to the massage giver. *Impetigo, ringworm, moles,* and *rashes* or *inflammation* are among the contagious skin disorders encountered.

Impetigo is a streptococcal infection of the skin characterized by small, fluid-filled blisters. Massage is contraindicated until the lesions have healed completely. Reddened ring-shaped scaly or blistered patches mark a contagious fungal infection, *ringworm*. Massage of the affected area is contraindicated due to possible spread of infection. Some *moles* may be contagious, especially if they are bleeding, open, or rough-edged. Avoid massaging over or near the site. A physician should examine the child with *skin rashes* or inflammation to determine the cause and whether the condition is contagious. Massage is contraindicated.

Orthopedic Conditions

In the case of an orthopedic condition, you should consult the child's physician to rule out the possibility of risk to bone or underlying tissues. The integrity of the bone and stage in the healing process are important considerations to discuss with a physician before massage.

Amputation. Generally, no massage should be given for at least 6 to 8 weeks to the area where the appendage has been removed. Massage should not be given over or near any openings in the skin, as infection may result.

Dislocation. *Subluxation* and *dislocation* of the hips are the most common types of bone displacement seen in children with special needs. Massage to the area is contraindicated—especially the more vigorous strokes. Massage is contraindicated for congenital dislocated hips (CDH), as it may interfere with the healing process.

Fracture. Massaging over the site of an unstable fracture may hinder the healing process and can create internal complications. Do not massage over the site of a break or rupture in a bone until it is well-healed. Massage using very gentle pressure then may be introduced, upon physician approval, to assist the recovery of the skin and lymphatic flow.

Osteoporosis. *Osteoporosis* is the decreasing of density and weight of bone, causing it to become brittle and fracture easily. Pain and deformity may occur. Factors in the development of osteoporosis include nutritional disturbances, calcium depletion, and decreased mobility (Nelson, 1996; Behrman, Kliegman, & Arvin, 1996). Some medications may also contribute to osteoporosis. Massage should not be given in the presence of osteoporosis. The child may enjoy simple, gentle touching from an adult's relaxed hand. This touch also may help reduce pain.

Osteogenesis Imperfecta (OI). Fractures and skeletal deformities characterize osteogenesis imperfecta. There are four types of OI with varying degrees of bone fragility and deformity. Some children with OI die as newborns. Others, who present with osteoporosis, bone brittleness, and occasional fractures, have a normal life expectancy (Nelson, 1996; Behrman, Kliegman, & Arvin, 1996). Consult the physician to assess the integrity of the child's bones before introducing massage. Very gentle stroking may be appropriate in mild cases; in more serious cases, only a relaxed hand placement is advised.

Abdominal Conditions

The presence of the following conditions in the abdominal cavity could be potential contraindications for massage. These conditions require medical intervention and would most likely be aggravated by massage.

Massage often is a beneficial treatment for constipation. However, the etiology of the constipation must be considered carefully, as there may be a structural blockage. Do not use massage if nausea, vomiting, or diarrhea is present; these may indicate signs of gastrointestinal infection. Although abdominal massage may not be indicated for the following conditions, it may be appropriate to massage other body parts, with physician approval.

Abdominal aortic aneurysm. An aneurysm is a sac or ballooning formed by the dilation of the wall of an artery—the abdominal aorta, in this case. Aneurysms are caused by the pressure of blood flowing through a weakened area. An abdominal aortic aneurysm is sometimes observed as a throbbing swelling. Abdominal massage must be avoided as it could rupture the aneurysm. The child's physician should be consulted about massage for other body parts. Medical attention is critical.

Abdominal distention, masses, or lumps. Abdominal distention or a mass may indicate a structural blockage or other serious medical condition. Medical attention is necessary.

Inguinal and abdominal hernia. *Herniation* involves the protrusion of the intestine through a weakened area of the inguinal canal or abdominal wall. This condition requires medical attention. Avoid abdominal massage. Pressure to the abdominal region may cause damage to the protruding organ.

Inflammatory Conditions

Massage is generally contraindicated when inflammation is present or if an anti-inflammatory medication is being taken, as it may irritate the joint space or tissues. This is particularly true of strokes that involve kneading or manipulation. Simple, gentle touching to offer comfort is indicated in this situation.

Acute inflammations. Some acute inflammations require immediate medical intervention. They include

- *encephalitis*—inflammation of the brain
- *meningitis*—inflammation of the membranes that cover the brain and spinal cord
- *peritonitis*—inflammation of the membrane that lines the wall of the abdomen and envelops the abdominal organs
- *appendicitis*—inflammation of the appendix

General massage is contraindicated until all signs of infection have passed. Upon physician approval, gentle stroking may help during recovery. Surgical sites should not be massaged until 6 to 8 weeks post surgery and only with a physician's approval.

Inflamed or very swollen joints. Avoid joints that are painful, swollen, or warm. Juvenile Rheumatoid Arthritis* (JRA) is a disease or group of diseases characterized by synovitis (chronic inflammation of the membrane lining the joint spaces) and other symptoms. The cause is unknown but hypothesized to result from an autoimmune reaction or infection with an unidentified microorganism (Nelson, 1996; Behrman, Kliegman, & Arvin, 1996). The appropriateness of massage depends on the type of JRA, the stage, and the presence of other symptoms. For example, general massage would be contraindicated if fever or rash were present. However, it may be used in the sub-acute phase to increase mobility and decrease stress and pain.

Neurological/Nervous System Conditions

Encephalitis and Meningitis have been previously discussed under inflammatory conditions.

Seizures are involuntary disturbances of brain function that may present as loss or impairment of consciousness, abnormal motor or behavioral activity, or disturbances of sensory or autonomic functioning. Massage is contraindicated during a seizure, as the adult's main concern should be to protect the child. However, massage at other times is considered appropriate. The adult should note if there is an increase in seizure activity during or following massage. If so, massage would be contraindicated; however, the child may benefit from other forms of touch.

Spinal Cord Injury* is damage to the spinal cord that results in loss of motor, some autonomic function, and sensation below the level of the injury. There may be partial or complete lesion. Massage may be indicated for children with spinal cord injuries if cautions are considered. Massage is contraindicated if there are blood clots. Extreme care should be used when massaging areas with impaired sensation. Each child will respond differently to gentle pressure. The massage giver must make sure that the touch is pleasurable and does not produce negative autonomic responses such as an increase in blood pressure, bradycardia, headache, or sweating.

Respiratory Conditions

Asthma* is a diffuse, obstructive lung disease with hyper-reactivity of the airways to different stimuli including allergens, respiratory infections, exercise, stress, and anxiety. Symptoms include wheezing, coughing, increased mucous production, rapid, shallow or labored breathing, and prolonged expiration (Nelson, 1996; Behrman, Kliegman, & Arvin, 1996). Although a full-body wellness massage is contraindicated while a child is having an asthma incident, children may find soothing touch to be comforting and calming while they receive their treatments (inhaler, nebulizer). It also can be calming to the adult who is helping the child manage the incident. Massage, deep breathing, and relaxation activities are helpful in the post-acute stage to encourage children to learn strategies to reduce anxiety before and during an incident.

Pneumonia is an inflammation of the lungs. Respiratory viruses are the most common cause of pneumonia in early childhood. Bacterial pneumonia is not as common during childhood, but tends to be a more severe infection. Non-infectious causes include aspiration of food or gastric acid, hypersensitivities, and others. Symptoms vary and may include runny or stuffy nose, cough, fever, and wheezing and difficulty breathing (Nelson, 1996; Behrman, Kliegman, & Arvin, 1996). Massage is contraindicated in the acute phase.

Digestive System Disorders

Hepatitis is an inflammation of the liver, producing symptoms that vary in severity, such as fatigue, jaundice, abdominal pain, nausea, and diarrhea. Hepatitis is usually caused by viral infection but also can be caused by exposure to toxins or drugs. Massage is contraindicated in the acute stage. The appropriateness of massage for those with chronic hepatitis depends on their overall health (Werner & Benjamin, 1998).

Jaundice is a symptom of liver or gall bladder dysfunction that occurs when there is an excess of bilirubin. The skin, eyes, and mucous membranes appear yellowish. Circulatory massage is contraindicated until the liver is fully functional (Werner & Benjamin, 1998).

Diabetes* (Juvenile-Onset Diabetes) is the most common endocrine-metabolic disorder in childhood and adolescence. It is a syndrome caused by a deficiency of insulin or its action, causing abnormal metabolism of carbohydrates, proteins, and fats. Children with diabetes are dependent on insulin (Nelson, 1996; Behrman, Kliegman, & Arvin, 1996). Massage may be appropriate with physician's approval for children with diabetes, if their insulin levels are stable, tissues are healthy, and there are no other cardiac, kidney, circulatory, sensation, or blood pressure contraindications. Rattray (1994) reported that it is possible for massage to destabilize a person with diabetes. Increased activity increases the uptake of insulin by the body, and it is thought that massage, which increases circulation, may affect the body in the same way.

Other Medical Concerns

This global category could accommodate a wide variety of disorders. Discussed here are some of the more common conditions. Any questions or concerns about a child's medical status and the appropriateness of massage should be directed to the child's physician.

Acquired Immune Deficiency Syndrome* (AIDS). AIDS is a disease of the immune system caused by infection by the human immunodeficiency virus (HIV). The infection leads to susceptibility to multiple infections that usually occur only in people with compromised immunity (Werner & Benjamin, 1998). Upon approval from the child's physician, very gentle massage may be beneficial to the infant or child with AIDS and their parent, especially from a psychosocial perspective. As the disease progresses, the massage giver may need to lighten the touch or simply hold the child's hands or feet.

Because the child's immune system is compromised, it is important that the massage giver be free of bacterial or viral infections that can be transmitted to the child. Be sure to follow the infection-control procedures of your facility regarding hand-washing and the use of gloves. To avoid risk of infection to the child or yourself, do not massage over areas of non-intact skin. Also avoid contact with other body fluids. Follow Universal Precautions as determined by the child's physician or the local health department. If the massage giver's skin is intact, thorough hand-washing before and after the massage should provide sufficient protection to the child and the interventionist.

Cancer. Cancer can be defined as the unrestrained growth of cells into tumors that invade tissues and organs and spread throughout the body (Clayman, 1989; Werner & Benjamin, 1998). In most cases, the exact cause of childhood cancer is unknown. It is believed that environmental and genetic factors are involved in the development of most cancers. But childhood cancers tend to develop in tissues that do not come in direct contact with the environment (Nelson, 1996; Behrman, Kliegman, & Arvin, 1996).

Consultation with the child's oncologist is necessary before providing massage. Some references recommend avoiding massage that enhances circulation. Consider alternate forms of touch and tactile input (e.g., gentle-touch pressure, swaddling, holding) to offer compassion, promote relaxation, and decrease pain. It is hoped that research will determine massage not to be only safe, but also beneficial to children and adults with cancer.

Cysts/foreign bodies. Avoid massage over the area of cysts or other foreign bodies—the bodies could rupture.

Gastroesphogeal reflux is the regurgitation of acid fluid from the stomach into the esophagus. Marcia Dunn Klein (personal communication, 1999) reported that children with reflux often are uncomfortable with abdominal massage. She recommended that children with reflux be positioned on a wedge when in supine. She also suggested that they be massaged before or at least 45 minutes after feeding.

Gastrointestinal or jejunostomy feeding tubes. The child's physician should be consulted about structural contraindications for abdominal massage. Generally, massage near the area should be avoided for 6 to 8 weeks after surgery. Be sure to avoid introducing oil near the skin opening that could cause infection. Take special care around the stoma site. Some children's tubes are dislodged more easily than others. Gentle hand placement on other areas of the abdomen, rather than traditional massage, is the safest approach. The child also may welcome massage to other parts of the body.

Recent surgery. A physician's approval for massage is *mandatory* after any type of surgery. Generally, massage should not be given on or near the area, for at least 6 to 8 weeks after surgery. Breaks or openings in the scars or sutures should not be massaged, as it could disrupt the healing process or cause infections. If endorsed by the physician, massage to other areas of the body may be very comforting.

Undiagnosed conditions or unusual tissue feel. If the child's skin or underlying tissues look or feel unusual, consult the physician before proceeding with the massage program.

Ventilators. If a child is on a ventilator, check with his or her physician to ascertain medical stability for tactile input.

Endangerment Sites

Endangerment sites or *sites of caution* are areas of the body that warrant caution because massage or deep pressure could cause damage to the underlying structures. Structures that may be at risk include nerves, blood vessels, organs, and lymph nodes.

Nerves can become impinged or compressed, causing pain or discomfort. Entrapment of an artery blocks the circulation. Occlusion of the major arteries of the neck (carotid) can cause the child to black out. Entrapment of a vein can injure the vessel and potentially create varicosities, hemorrhages, or clots. The kidneys are only partially protected by the rib cage, and therefore, percussion to the upper lumbar area can cause damage. On the back, one should avoid pressing the paraspinal muscles in toward the spinous processes that may cause pain.

The colon can become pinned during deep-stomach massage. Abdominal massage should move in a clockwise direction to assist the movement of fecal material. Lymph nodes may be inflamed if the child has an infection, and they should not be massaged.

When massaging children, one should *never* use a strong enough pressure to cause damage, but the massage giver should be well-aware of the anatomical location of these sites of caution. Endangerment sites vary among different references. The massage giver should use lighter pressure or avoid the following areas:

- Orbital (eyes)

- Anterior triangle of the neck (front of the neck and throat)

- Posterior aspect of the neck (back of the neck)

- Axilla (armpit)

- Brachial region (medial aspect of the upper arm)

- Cubital area (front of the elbow)

- Near olecranon process (back of elbow/funny bone)

- Upper lumbar (mid-back/kidney area)

- Umbilical area (naval)

- Femoral triangle (inner upper leg)

- Popliteal fossa (back of the knee)

- Inguinal area (groin)

Medical Contraindications for Massage

Note: These contraindications have been compiled from a variety of resources in the literature. This is meant to represent the general consensus regarding contraindications. Any specific concerns should always be presented to the attending physician.

Massage is totally contraindicated	Massage is contraindicated at a particular site	Type of massage depends of stage of disease or condition
Aortic aneurysm	Abdominal mass, lump or distention	Aids
Appendicitis (acute)	Burns (unhealed)	Asthma
Certain cardiac conditions	Cysts or foreign bodies	Cancer
Edema due to heart decompensation and/or kidney problems	Dislocation	Diabetes
Encephalitis	Fractures (unhealed)	Seizures
Hemophilia	G-tubes	Spinal cord injury
Hepatitis	Hematomas (acute)	
Infection–with fever and pain	Hernias	
Jaundice/hyperbilirubinemia	Inflammatory conditions (acute and early sub acute)	
Lymphagitis	Nausea, vomiting, reflux, or diarrhea	
Osteogenesis imperfecta	Open wounds	
Osteomyelitis or septic arthritis	Recent surgery (may proceed with physician approval after 6–8 weeks post surgery)	
Osteoporosis		
Peritonitis (acute)	Rheumatoid arthritis and acute osteoarthritis (acute)	
Phlebitis (acute)	Skin conditions–allergies, warts, etc.	
Pneumonia (acute)	Synovitis	
Skin diseases, including infectious diseases, scabies, lice, fleas	Varicose veins	
Thrombosis		
Tuberculosis		
Undiagnosed conditions		
Unusual tissue feel		
Very high blood pressure		

Summary

To prevent transmitting disease to or from the child, always wash your hands thoroughly before and after the massage. Some practitioners feel that washing their hands also helps them mentally release negative energy or stress they may have assumed from the recipient during the massage process. Done carefully, after a consultation with the child's physician, massage generally is a safe and comforting technique. The experience offers many physical and emotional benefits to the child and his or her parents.

Below is a sample approval form for pediatric massage that can be presented to physicians. It may be copied for your professional use. You may need to consult your legal department regarding specific guidelines for your facility.

Sample Physician Approval Form
for Pediatric Massage

LETTERHEAD

PHYSICIAN APPROVAL FOR PEDIATRIC MASSAGE

Child's Name: _____ Date of Birth: _____

Diagnosis: _____

_____

Physician: _____

Please check one of the following:

_____ This child may participate in a pediatric massage program, which may increase circulation.

_____ This child should not receive massage.

_____ This child may participate in a pediatric massage program with the following limitations:

_____

_____

_____

Please indicate if the child has any conditions for which massage would be contraindicated.

_____

_____

_____

_____
Physician's Signature

_____
Approval Date

Sample Letter to Physician or Primary Health Care Provider

Dear Dr. _____:

Your patient, Shana, has been referred to me by her physical therapist for a pediatric massage consult and parent instruction. I would like to ask for your approval of her participation. I am enclosing a form for your input and signature.

I am a pediatric occupational therapist and certified infant massage instructor. For more than 15 years, I have been sharing massage with families with children who have special needs and have found it to be a very positive experience.

Shana's mother and therapist are interested in using massage to enhance Shana's body awareness, symmetry, and organization. They also would like to use it as a general method of calming and pain reduction.

As I'm sure you are aware, there are many other benefits of massage when adapted to respond to the child's behavioral and physiological cues. They may include better attainment of the quiet alert state to maximize feeding and interaction; improved circulation; improved parent-child interaction; increased parental confidence; deeper respiration; increased quiet sleep periods; and enhanced gastrointestinal functioning.

The goals, techniques, and benefits are highly individualized. For some children who are highly sensitive or fragile, we start with just a gentle hand placement, with the goal of eventually being able to use stroking. I am sending a copy of a research article and would be happy to provide more information if you would like.

Pending your approval, we have arranged to teach Michelle, Shana's mother, the massage techniques with Shana at her home on September 15. We plan to videotape the session for Michelle to keep and review. She also will be given written materials with illustrations describing the strokes. I am sure that Michelle and Shana will enjoy the massage and feel comfortable with the techniques. We will schedule additional sessions to modify the massage as needed.

If you have any questions, please feel free to contact me at the phone number above. If you agree to this plan, please complete and sign the enclosed form and return it to me. Thank you very much. I am looking forward to sharing pediatric massage with Shana and Michelle.

Sincerely,

Chapter 8

Introduction

A significant body of research supports the clinical findings of massage benefits to infants and children. Since 1991 when *Pediatric Massage* (Fuhr & Drehobl, 1991) was published, an enormous amount of research has been conducted to further validate the powerful role of therapeutic touch and massage. Initial research in the area of infant massage primarily addressed preterm infants in the hospital setting. Current literature explores the role of massage with varying populations, ages, and diagnostic categories.

It is very difficult to provide *only* tactile input when working with infants and children. Many of the studies used a combination of tactile and kinesthetic stimulation or tactile and vestibular stimulation. Auditory and visual stimulation occurred naturally as components of an interactive massage or touch experience.

Baseline and outcome measurements varied between studies, as did the specific techniques used, the frequency and duration of intervention, the sample size, and the health and developmental status of the subjects. Parent involvement is another important variable in a number of the studies. It is difficult to ascertain whether the positive effects evidenced in some of the studies were due to increased parent interaction, the tactile/kinesthetic or tactile/vestibular stimulation, or other factors.

Because of the controlled nature of research, most of the studies used standardized treatment protocols. The treatment programs generally did not address individualization or responsivity to infant cues, temperament, neurobehavioral organization, or self-regulatory competence. In practice, however, an interactive massage varies with each individual in terms of the type and location of touch, length of treatment, positioning, and response of the infant or child.

The purpose of this research chart is to present a sampling of studies most applicable to pediatrics. Refer to the full text articles as cited in the References for more specific information about the design, implementation, and outcome of each study.

Subjects	**ADHD**
	28 adolescents with Attention Deficit/Hyperactivity Disorder
Year	1998
Investigator(s)	Field, T.; Quintino, O.; Hernandez-Reif, M.; Koslovsky, G.
Conditions	The experimental group received massage therapy and the control group received relaxation therapy for 10 consecutive school days.
Results	Following the sessions, the massage therapy group (but not the relaxation therapy group) rated themselves as happier. Observers rated them as fidgeting less.
	After the 2-week period, their teachers reported more time on task and assigned them lower hyperactivity scores based on classroom behavior.

Subjects	**Arthritis**
	20 children age 5.4 to 14.8 years old with mild to moderate juvenile rheumatoid arthritis
Year	1997
Investigator(s)	Field, T.; Hernadez-Reif, M.; Seligman, S.; Krasnegor, J.; Sunshine, W.; Rivas-Chacon, R.; Schaunberg, S.; Kuhn, C.
Conditions	Children in the experimental group were massaged by their parents 15 minutes a day for 30 days.
	Children in the control group used relaxation therapy.
Results	Immediately after massage, the children in the experimental group showed

- decreased anxiety and
- decreased cortisol levels.

During the 30-day study period, their pain decreased as measured by self-report, parent report, and physician assessment. Parents reported less pain-limiting of vigorous activity. A decrease in parental anxiety was reported for those giving massage.

Subjects	**Asthma**
	32 children with asthma, ranging from 4 to 14 years of age
Year	1998
Investigator(s)	Field, T.; Henteleff, T.; Hernadez-Reif, M.; Martinez, E.; Mavunda, K.; Kuhn, C.; Schanberg, C.

Conditions	Sixteen 4 to 8 year-olds (Group A) and sixteen 9 to 14 year-olds (Group B) were randomly selected to receive either massage or relaxation therapy.
	Children in the massage therapy group received 20 minutes of massage from their parents every night for 30 days.
	Children in the relaxation therapy group used progressive muscle relaxation with their parents for 20 minutes every night for 30 days.
Results	Younger children (Group A) who received massage therapy showed

- an immediate decrease in behavioral anxiety and cortisol levels,
- an improvement in their attitude toward asthma, and
- an improved peak air flow and other pulmonary functions.

Older children (Group B) who received massage therapy

- reported lower anxiety,
- showed improvement in their attitude toward asthma, and
- showed only one measure of pulmonary functioning improved.

Subjects	**Autism**
	22 preschool children with autism who attended a special preschool
Year	1996
Investigator(s)	Field, T.; Lasko, D.; Mundy, P.; Henteleff, T.; Kabat, S.; Talpins, S.; Dowling, M.
Conditions	Children in the treatment group received touch therapy (massage through clothing) from a volunteer student for 15 minutes a day, 2 days a week for 4 weeks.
	In the touch control group, a volunteer held each child and engaged the child in a game for the same time period.
Results	Touch aversion and off-task behavior decreased in both groups.
	Orienting to irrelevant sounds and stereotypic behaviors decreased in both groups but significantly more in the touch-therapy group.
	Children in the touch-therapy group also made significant improvements on the Autism Behavioral Checklist (Krug, Arick, & Almond, 1979) and the Early Social Communication Scales, including social relating and joint attention.

Subjects	**Child and adolescent psychiatric patients with anxiety**
	52 hospitalized children and adolescents with depression and adjustment disorders

Year	1992
Investigator(s)	Field, T.; Morrow, C.; Valdeon, C.; Larson, S.; Kuhn, C.; Schanberg, S.
Conditions	Subjects in the experimental group received a daily, 30-minute back massage for 5 days.
	Subjects in the control group viewed relaxing videotapes only.
Results	After massage, subjects in the experimental group were less depressed and anxious and had lower saliva cortisol.
	Nurses rated the massage-group subjects on the last day of the study as less anxious and more cooperative.

Additional findings:

- Nighttime sleep increased over this period.
- Urinary cortisol and norepinephrine levels decreased, but only for the depressed subjects

---

Subjects	**Cystic Fibrosis**
	20 children 5 to 12 years of age with cystic fibrosis
Year	1999
Investigator(s)	Hernandez-Reif, M.; Field, T.; Krasnegor, J.; Martinez, E.; Schwartzman, M.; Mavunda, K.
Conditions	Each child in treatment group received a 20-minute massage from a parent every night at bedtime for one month.
	A parent read to each child in the control group for the same amount of time.
Results	Parents and children in the massage group reported reduced anxiety after the first and last session.
	Mood and peak air-flow readings also improved for children in the massage therapy group.

Subjects	**Dermatitis**
	Children with atopic dermatitis
Year	1998
Investigator(s)	Schachner, L.; Field, T.; Hernandez-Reif, M.; Duarte, A. M.; Krasnegor, J.
Conditions	Children in the experimental group were given standard topical care and massage by their parents for 20 minutes a day for 1 month.
	Children in the control group received standard topical care only.

Results	Parents of massaged children reported lower anxiety levels. Children improved on clinical measures including redness, scaling, lichenification, excoriation, and puritis.
	Children in the control group only improved on the scaling measure.

Subjects	**Diabetes**
	20 children with diabetes
Year	1997
Investigator(s)	Field, T.; Hernandez-Reif, M.; LaGreca A.; Shaw, K.; Schanberg, S.; Kuhn, C.
Conditions	Children in the treatment group received 20 minutes of massage daily from a parent before bedtime for 30 days.
	Children in the control group received relaxation therapy from a parent for the same amount of time.
Results	The massage groups' immediate effects were
	• reduced parent anxiety and depression, and
	• reduced child anxiety, fidgeting, and depressed affect.
	Over the 30-day period, compliance for insulin and food regulation improved, and blood-glucose levels decreased to the normal range.

Subjects	**Fathers and babies**
	32 Australian firstborn babies and their fathers
Year	1992
Investigator(s)	Scholtz, K.; Samuels, C.
Conditions	Australian families with first-born babies were studied, for the effects of a 4-week postpartum training program (demonstration of baby massage and the Burleigh Relaxation Bath technique), with emphasis on the father-infant relationship. The treatment group consisted of 16 families that were assigned to the treatment group, and 16 families that served as controls.
Results	During the 12-week home observation, treatment-group infants greeted their fathers with more eye contact, smiling, vocalizing, reaching, and orienting responses, and showed less avoidance behaviors. In a 10-minute observation, the treatment-group fathers showed greater involvement with their infants.

Subjects	**HIV**
	28 neonates born to HIV-positive mothers

Year	1996
Investigator(s)	Scafidi, F.; Field, T.
Conditions	Infants in the treatment group received three 15-minute massages daily for 10 weekdays.
	Infants in the control group received the standard care.
Results	Massaged infants showed

- greater daily weight gain at the end of the treatment period
- superior performance on most of the Brazelton newborn cluster scores

The control group showed declining performance.

Subjects	**Maternal Depression**
	40 1- to 3-month old infants born to depressed, adolescent mothers of low socio-economic status
Year	1996
Investigator(s)	Field, T.; Grizzle, N.; Scafidi, F.; Abrams, S.; Richardson, S.
Conditions	Infants in the experimental group received 15 minutes of massage 2 days a week for a 6-week period.
	Infants in the control group were rocked during the same period.
Results	The infants who experienced massage therapy

* spent more time in active alert and active awake states,
* cried less, and
* had lower salivary cortisol levels (suggesting lower stress).

After the massage (versus the rocking sessions), the infants spent less time in an active awake state, suggesting that massage may be more effective than rocking for inducing sleep.

Over the 6-week period, the massage-therapy infants

- gained more weight,
- showed greater improvement on emotionality, sociability, and soothability temperament dimensions, and
- had greater decreases in urinary stress catecholamines/hormones (norepinephrine, epinephrine, cortisol).

Subjects	**Motoric Impairment**
	19 infants diagnosed with motor delay or neuro-motor deficit, attending an early intervention program with their mothers

Age: 3–19 months at the beginning of the study

None of the infants had moderate or severe sensory impairment of hearing or vision.

Year	1988
Investigator(s)	Hansen, R.; Ulrey, G.
Conditions	Infants in the experimental group received Leboyer infant massage in addition to their regular sensory motor activities.
	Infants in the control group received the regular program for early intervention that provided parents with sensory motor activities.
Results	Both the control and experimental groups progressed in the child and parent cueing, contact, and organization behaviors or an attachment-separation-individuation observation protocol.
	Infants in the experimental group showed significantly more progress when the total child and parent behaviors were combined. Only the experimental group showed significant change in the caregiver-infant discrepancy score.
	Results suggested that the handling procedures may have facilitated the development of more compatible and positive interactions between caregivers and their infants.
	There was no statistically significant change in mental or motor functioning status of either group on the *Bayley Scales of Infant Development* (Bayley, 1969).

Subjects	**Post-Traumatic Stress Disorder**
	60 1st through 5th graders who showed classroom behavior problems after Hurricane Andrew
Year	1996
Investigator(s)	Field, T.; Seligman, S.; Scafidi, F.; Schanberg, S.
Conditions	These children were randomly assigned to a massage-therapy (MT) or a video-attention (VA) group. Scores on the Post-Traumatic Stress Disorder Index suggest the subjects were experiencing severe post-traumatic stress.
Results	Subjects who received MT reported being happier and less anxious and had lower salivary cortisol levels after the therapy than VA subjects. The MT group subjects showed more sustained changes as manifested by lower scores for anxiety, depression, and self-drawings. MT subjects also were observed to be more relaxed.

Subjects	**Prematurity**
	30 preterm infants who were hospitalized in a Level III NICU
	Gestational age: 26 to 32 weeks at birth
Year	1996
Investigator(s)	Harrison, L.; Olivet, L.; Cunningham, K.; Bodin, M.; Hicks, C.
Conditions	Infants in the experimental group received 15 minutes of gentle human touch (GHT) each day for 5 days, beginning when they were between 6 to 9 days of age.
	The researcher gently placed one hand on the infant's head and the other across the infant's lower back and buttocks. GHT avoided touch to the chest and abdomen. Touch was maintained for 15 minutes.
	Infants in the control group received the amount of touch associated with usual NICU care.
Results	No significant difference in oxygen saturation or heart-rate levels before, during, or after GHT periods.
	No significant difference in the percentage of quiet sleep, compared with baseline, touch, and post-touch periods.
	Significantly less active sleep during periods of GHT, compared with baseline and post-touch periods.
	Less motor activity and behavioral distress during GHT sessions than during baseline or post-touch periods.
	Infants in the experimental group spent more days receiving phototherapy.
	No differences were found between infants in the experimental and control groups on the number of days on supplemental oxygen, weight gain, or scores on the Brazelton Neonatal Behavioral Assessment Scale.
	A 15-minute GHT intervention has no adverse effect on heart rate or oxygen-saturation levels. GHT seems to have a soothing effect.

Subjects	**Prematurity**
	11 stable preterm boys
	Gestational age: 23–34 weeks
	Birth weight = 630–2180 grams
	Postnatal age was 4 to 132 days
	Six infants were receiving supplemental oxygen.

Year	1993
Investigator(s)	Acolet, D.; Modi, N.; Giannakoulopoulos, X.; Bond, C.; Weg, W.; Clow, A.; Glover, V.
Conditions	Gentle massage of the trunk and limbs, lasting about 20 minutes and using arachis oil, was given by a nurse.
	Infants in the control group provided blood samples at the same time of day and over the same time interval.
Results	There was no significant change in oxygenation or oxygen requirement before, during, and after massage.
	There was a slight decrease in skin temperature.
	The infants receiving massage showed a consistent decrease in plasma cortisol concentrations. (The stress of pain results in an increase in cortisol concentrations.)

Subjects	**Prematurity**
	40 preterm infants from intermediate care unit
	Mean gestational age: 30 weeks
	Mean birth weight: 1176 grams
Year	1990
Investigator(s)	Scafidi, F.; Field, T.; Schanberg, S.
	(Replicated an earlier study by Scafidi, et al)
Conditions	Treatment infants received tactile/kinesthetic stimulation for three 15-minute periods during 3 consecutive hours per day for 10 weekdays.
	Infants in the control group received standard nursery care.
Results	The treatment group infants averaged a 21% greater weight gain per day and were discharged 5 days earlier.
	The treatment group performance was superior on the habituation cluster items of the Brazelton scale.
	The infants in the treatment group were more active during the stimulation sessions than the observation sessions.
	There were no significant differences in sleep/wake states and activity levels between the groups.

Subjects	**Prematurity**
	21 healthy preterm infants
	Gestational age: 32 to 36 weeks

Year	1989
Investigator(s)	Strong, C.
Conditions	Infants were observed for 50 minutes as a baseline. Treatment was a 10-minute back massage. The infants were then observed post-treatment for 50 minutes.
Results	Younger infants had a decrease in pulse and increase in respiratory rate after massage, as compared with the baseline.
	Older infants showed an increase in pulse immediately after massage.
	All age groups showed a decrease in stress-related behavior during the first 10 minutes after massage and an increase in frequency of self-comforting behavior after massage.
	The infants also spent more time in quiet sleep after massage than before. There was a trend for infants of all ages to take less time to console themselves after having a massage than before.
	None of the observed differences were statistically significant.

Subjects	**Prematurity**
	36 preterm infants and their parents
	Mean gestational age at birth: 29.6 weeks
	Mean birth weight: 1337grams
	None of the infants had congenital anomalies or had undergone surgery.
Year	1989
Investigator(s)	Harrison, L.; Leeper, J.; Yoon, M.
Conditions	Infants were monitored during parent visits. No limits were imposed on the type of touch the parents could provide.
	Infants and parents were videotaped during parent visits to the NICU when the infants were 5–14 days of age. Parents were encouraged to interact with their infants as usual.
	Videotapes were coded to describe the physical characteristics of parent touch. This was paired with the infants' physiologic data at the time of parent touch.
Results	The number of abnormal oxygen saturation levels increased during periods of parent touch, however, the analysis of individual infants indicated that some infants responded more favorably to parent touch with increased mean oxygen saturation levels and a decrease in the percentage of abnormal oxygen saturation values.
	Variability in the effects of parent touch on infant heart rate also

was seen, but there were very few abnormal heart rate values observed. Heart rate was less affected by parent touch than oxygen saturation.

Subjects	**Prematurity**
	33 healthy, premature infants
	Mean gestational age upon entry to study: 35 weeks
	Mean birth weight: 1431.9 grams for controls and 1470 grams for experimental group
Year	1988
Investigator(s)	White-Traut, R.; Goldman, M. B.
Conditions	Infants in the treatment group received Rice Infant Sensorimotor Stimulation Technique (RISS) when infant weight was 1750 grams.
	Treatment was given once a day for 15 minutes for 10 days or until discharge whichever came first. (See Rice, 1979 for further description.)
	Infants in the control group received routine nursery care.
Results	**Body temperature.** No significant difference between the groups at baseline and two post-treatment times.
	Heart rate. At baseline, there was no significant difference between the groups. At 8 minutes, the control group was slightly lower than baseline and the treatment group was higher than baseline. At 15 and 20 minutes, there was no significant difference between the groups.
	Respiration rate. At baseline there was no significant difference between the groups. At 8 minutes the control group was slightly higher than baseline and the treatment group was higher than the control group. At 15 and 20 minutes there was no significant difference between the groups.
	Changes in body temperature, respiration and heart rate were within acceptable limits.

Subjects	**Prematurity**
	33 healthy preterm infants and their mothers
	Gestational age: 28–35 weeks
	Birth weight: appropriate for gestational age
Year	1988
Investigator(s)	White-Traut, R.; Nelson, M.
Conditions	The infants and their mothers were placed in one of 3 groups:

Group A—Routine nursery care

Group B—Unstructured talking (mothers sang or talked to their infants for 15 minutes)

Group C—Rice Infant Sensorimotor Stimulation Technique (RISS). See Rice, 1979 for further description.

Treatment occurred during four time intervals between 24–72 hours after birth.

Results

Infants in RISS treatment achieved quiet alert state 80% of the time after treatment.

Mothers in the RISS group received significantly higher maternal-infant interaction scores.

There was a significant difference between the control group and the talk group in maternal sensitivity toward the infant and cognitive growth-fostering behavior.

Infants in the RISS and talk treatment groups scored higher on the Nursing Child Assessment Feeding Scale (NCAFS) than infants in the control group.

The talk and RISS groups differed little with regard to infant behaviors, but a large difference on the infant scale was seen between the routine care group and the talking group.

Subjects

Prematurity

50 healthy preterm infants

Gestational age: 28 to 36 weeks

Year

1987

Investigator(s)

Fernandez, A.; Patkar, S.; Chawla, C.; Taskar, T.; Prabhu, S.V.

Conditions

Babies in the experimental group had corn oil applied all over their bodies with a cotton swab. These babies were kept uncovered in the cradles on polyethylene sheets to prevent the oil from rubbing off. Oil applications were repeated every 4 hours during a 72-hour period.

Control babies and experimental babies were kept in open cradles equipped with a radiant lamp. The temperature of all babies was measured every 2 hours. If the infant's temperature was below 37° C, the lamp was turned on. If the temperature was above 37.6° C, the lamp was turned off.

Results

The babies in the experimental group required much less use of the warmer to maintain their body temperature, compared with the control group, regardless of gestational weight.

Infants in the experimental group showed a marked increase in serum triglycerides, indicating that oil gets absorbed through the skin of preterm babies and acts as a source of nutrition to the babies.

Subjects	**Prematurity**
	33 healthy, preterm infants
	Mean gestational age at time of study: 35 weeks
	Mean birth weight of controls: 1431 grams
	Mean birth weight of experimental infants: 1472.4 grams
Year	1987
Investigator(s)	White-Traut, R.; Pate, C.
Conditions	Subjects in the treatment group received Rice Infant Sensorimotor Stimulation Technique (RISS) when each infant's weight was 1750 grams.
	Treatment was given once a day for 15 minutes for 10 days or until discharge, whichever came first. (See Rice, 1979 for further description.)
	Infants in the control group received routine nursery care.
Results	At baseline, there was no significant difference in infant state between the 2 groups. Eighty percent of the infants were in one of the two sleep states.

At mid-treatment:

- 31% of the treatment group was in the quiet alert state versus 4.8% of the control group.

- 22.5% of the treatment group was in the active alert state versus 5.6% in the control group.

Immediately post-treatment:

- 58.4% of the treatment group was in the quiet alert state versus 1.6% of the control group.

- 4.2 % of treatment group was in the active alert state versus 8% of the control group.

At 5 minutes post-treatment:

- 36% of the treatment group was in the quiet alert state versus 1.5% of control group.

- 14% of the treatment group was in active alert state versus 5.6% of control group.

The RISS technique was successful in helping the infant organize his or her behavior state to achieve the quiet alert state.

Subjects	**Prematurity**

40 preterm, medically stable, neonates in the grower transitional nursery.

Mean gestational age: 31 weeks

Mean birth weight: 1,280 grams

Year	1986
Investigator(s)	Field, T.; Schanberg, S.; Scafidi, F.; Bauer, C.; Vega-Lahr, N.; Garcia, R.; Nystrom, J.; Kuhn, C.
Conditions	Infants in the treatment group received tactile/kinesthetic stimulation for three 15-minute periods at the beginning of three consecutive hours for 10 weekdays.

Infants in the control group received standard nursery care.

Results	The treatment group

- averaged 47% greater weight gain per day than the control group,

- was more active and alert during sleep/wake behavior observations, compared with the control group, and

- showed more mature habituation, orientation, motor skills, and range of state behavior on the Brazelton scale than the control group.

The treatment group's hospital stay was 6 days shorter, yielding a cost savings of about $3,000 per infant.

Subjects	**Prematurity**

36 stable premature infants

Gestational age: between 29–35 weeks

Birth weight: less than 1800 grams

Year	1986
Investigator(s)	White-Traut, R.; Tubeszewski, K.
Conditions	Subjects in the treatment group received Rice Infant Sensorimotor Stimulation Technique (RISS) when the infant's weight was 1750 grams.

Treatment was given once a day for 15 minutes for 10 days or until discharge, whichever came first. (See Rice, 1979 for further description.)

Infants in the control group received routine nursery care.

Results	Infants in the treatment group showed a trend toward greater weight gain and shorter duration of hospitalization, although not significantly different.
	There were no significant adverse physiologic effects.

Subjects	**Prematurity**
	15 preterm infants of 26–30 weeks post-conception age
	Mean gestational age: 28 weeks
	Birth weight: 720–1450 grams
	Infants were categorized as well, moderately ill, or sick.
Year	1985
Investigator(s)	Oehler, J.
Conditions	Each treatment session began with 80 seconds of no stimulation given. Three 80-second periods of stimulation were alternated with 80 seconds of undisturbed periods that followed.
	Three types of treatment were presented:
	• talking,
	• troking, and
	• talking plus stroking.
Results	Well infants had significantly more smiles and hand-to-mouth activity than the other groups during all three types of treatment.
	Sick infants had significantly more avoidance signals. Sick infants also showed the most avoidance during the combination of talking and touching.
	There were no significant changes in heart rate for any stimulus condition.

Subjects	**Prematurity**
	26 mechanically ventilated preterm infants, diagnosed with respiratory distress syndrome.
	Gestational age: 27–32 weeks
	Birth weight: at least 1000 grams
Year	1982
Investigator(s)	Jay, S.

Conditions	The 13 infants in the treatment group received 48 minutes of tactile contact each day. This consisted of 12 minutes of contact, four times daily for 10 days. Tactile contact was a gentle placement of the researcher's hand on the infant's head and abdomen. Thirteen infants served as a matched control group.
Results	The results indicated that very gentle human touch did not seem to *harm* the infants.
	No incidence of temperature drop, apnea, or seizure activity occurred during the touch periods. (Statistically, more incidences of apnea occurred in the treatment group; this was due to one infant.)
	No significant differences between the groups were reported in the areas of weight gain or loss, temperature stability, bradycardia, and advancement to or toleration of oral nutrients.
	Differences between the length of hospitalization of the two groups were invalid due to confounding variables.
	During the course of the study, oxygen requirements were consistently lower, hematocrit levels were higher, and there were fewer blood transfusions required in the treatment group.

Subjects	**Prematurity**
	40 preterm infants
	Birth weight: 1000–2000 grams
Year	1981
Investigator(s)	Rausch, P.
Conditions	Infants in the treatment group received three, 5-minute phases of tactile/kinesthetic treatment once a day for 10 days. Phases 1 and 3 consisted of gentle stroking. Phase 2 was gentle flexion and extension of the arms and legs.
	Infants in the control group received standard nursery care.
	Parents of subjects in both groups were encouraged to visit and handle their infants.
Results	The treatment group demonstrated
	• greater weight gain (the difference between groups was not statistically significant),
	• increased feeding intake, and
	• increased frequency of stooling.

Subjects	**Prematurity**
	30 premature infants
	Gestation: 32–37 weeks or less
	Birth weight: 1420–2245 grams
	Mothers of the infants were of low socio-economic status.
	The average hospital stay was 10 days.
Year	1979
Investigator(s)	Rice, R.
Conditions	Treatment occurred at home after hospital discharge.
	The mother administered the stroking treatment for 15 minutes, four times daily for 30 days. The stroking was followed by 5 minutes of rocking, holding, and cuddling.
	Infants in the treatment and control groups received regular visits from public health nurses who provided social reinforcement for appropriate mothering.
Results	The results indicated
	• significantly greater weight gain in the treatment group,
	• no significant difference in length of the body or head circumference, and
	• significantly greater mean appearance of the Landau and the labyrinthine head righting reflexes among the experimental group.
	The presence of these reflexes suggests greater neurological maturation at 4 months of age.

Subjects	**Prematurity**
	14 premature infants
	Gestational age: less than 38 weeks (mean: 33 weeks)
	Weight: 1800 grams or less. (The mean was 1441 for experimental infants and 1418 for controls.)
Year	1975
Investigator(s)	Kramer, M.; Chamorro, I.; Green, D.; Knutson, F.
Conditions	Infants in the treatment group received 48 minutes of tactile stimulation (gentle, nonrhythmic stroking) above the usual amount provided to preterm infants, for 2 weeks. Intervention was given before and after feeding.

Infants in the control group received routine nursery care.

Results	Infants in the treatment group exhibited more quiescence and increased rate of social development.
	Infants in both groups demonstrated good weight gain. There was no statistical difference between the groups, in weight gain or plasma cortisol levels in response to stress.

Subjects	**Prematurity**
	12 premature infants
	Gestational age: 36 weeks or less
	Birth weight: 1588–2041 grams
Year	1975
Investigator(s)	White, J.; Labarba, R.
Conditions	Infants in the treatment group received 15 minutes of input every 4 hours, above routine nursery care. Treatment was given on the 2nd through the 11th day of life.
	Treatment input consisted of rubbing the infants' neck, shoulders, legs, chest, and back, and flexing of the arms and legs.
	Infants in the control group received routine nursery care.
Results	Treatment group showed better weight gain and greater intake of formula with fewer feedings.
	There were no differences between the groups in body temperature, respiration, heart rate, and frequency of stooling and voiding.

Subjects	**Preschoolers**
	Typical preschool children
Year	1996
Investigator(s)	Field, T.; Kilmer, T.; Hernandez-Reif, M.; Burman, I.
Conditions	Preschool children received 20-minute massages twice a week for 5 weeks.
	The control group consisted of children on the wait list.
Results	Compared with the control group, the massaged children

- had better behavior ratings on state, vocalization, activity, and cooperation after the massage sessions on the first and last days of the study;

- were rated more optimally by their teachers at the end of the study;

- were rated by their parents as having less touch aversion and being more extroverted at the end of the study; and

- had a shorter latency to naptime by the end of the study.

Subjects	**Self-injurious behavior**
	One 14-year old girl diagnosed with Cornelia de Lange Syndrome, presenting with severe self-injurious behavior over 10 years of inpatient care
Year	1991
Investigator(s)	Dosseter, D.; Couryer, S.; Nicol, A.
Conditions	A nurse provided individual attention and massage using cream or oil for 30 minutes twice a day after a bath.
Results	The subject enjoyed and relaxed with massage from the first day. On the 3rd day, she wanted to massage the nurse.

Over the next 3 months, improvement was indicated by healing wounds and increased time without protective helmet and splints, decreased temper tantrums, and a gradual weaning from tranquilizers.

After 6 months

- no medications were needed for the first time in 10 years,

- no splints or helmet were needed, and

- all injuries had healed.

This improvement was maintained for 18 months with only a few mild and transient relapses.

Subjects	**SIDS Risk**
	23 caregiver-infant dyads receiving home-based services. Infants were at high risk for Sudden Infant Death Syndrome.
Year	1996
Investigator(s)	Pardew, E. M.
	Doctoral Dissertation
Conditions	Both groups received intensive home-based nursing service. The treatment group also received training in infant massage.
Results	Intensive home-based nursing services, which included infant massage, suggested a positive effect on the infant-caregiver interaction during routine feeding. Caregivers were unanimous in their satisfaction with infant massage instruction.

There are many studies that offered excellent data, as well as several published literature reviews, that are referenced in the Bibliography. Knowledge of past and current research, with an understanding of cultural and historical practice, is helpful when discussing massage with medical personnel. As with the area of pediatric care, pediatric massage continues to be a work in progress. All researchers are to be congratulated on their efforts in contributing to this body of knowledge.

Chapter **9**

Some Common Questions

How many times should I repeat a stroke?

There is not a set number of strokes. The best approach is to monitor the child's responses and select strokes that bring organization and pleasure. Later, you will be able to increase the variety of body parts you massage and the strokes you use. It is important to monitor the child's behavior before, during, and after massage to determine the overall effectiveness. The length of the massage also will depend on the age and medical fragility of the child. In a young infant, these cues will be more subtle. (Refer to Chapters 4 and 6 for more information.)

What precautions should I take for gastrostomy or jejunostomy tubes?

Always consult the child's physician before initiating massage. If there is no overt inflammation and the tube appears to be secure, you may be able to introduce gentle, circular stroking around the area, or just keep a hand on the stomach. Due to tube placement, children often get little input to this area, with the exception of feeding. **No lubrication** should be applied around the stoma site due to the chance of infection. (See Chapter 7 for specific information about massage when gastronomy or jejunostomy tubes are present.)

When should I massage the child?

The quiet alert state is ideal for optimal interaction. It is important that the massage fit into the daily routine to assure consistent follow-through. After a bath or during diaper changing is an ideal time as the child is already undressed. For older children, one may find that massage is helpful during stressful transitions or as a part of a regular sensory diet. Some children may benefit from being massaged in the morning to help in arousal and preparation for their day. Others may need massage after bathtime to help them transition to bedtime. Many older children will ask for massage if needed, if they perceive it as calming and helpful to their bodies. (See Chapter 4 for more information about the quiet alert state. See Chapter 3 for more information on sensory diet.)

How often should the child be massaged?

There is no set number. Once a day in some form is nice for continuity. Some parents find that it works best for their schedule to give a brief massage several times a day during dressing or diapering time. Massage also may be used throughout the day for transition times such as waking up, helping the child to attend, winding down from school, and transition to bedtime. Bear in mind that massage is not always used for relaxation; it also can help promote arousal and attention.

When is it appropriate to integrate massage into a therapy/educational program?

It's best to establish a therapeutic relationship with child and parent *before* introducing massage. Introduce massage after treatment goals have been established and there is a level of rapport with the family. Strokes should be introduced in a graded manner, allowing time for practice between therapy sessions. Education regarding handling and positioning can be incorporated along with the strokes. It also is important to note that in educational settings, children may not be disrobed. In any setting, removal of clothing is up to the discretion of the parents and child. Many strokes may be done over clothing or to body parts that are exposed such as the hands, feet, or face.

Are these massage techniques just for infants?

No! These strokes can be used with children up to 10 or 11 years of age, depending on the size of the child. At that point, extremities often become too large to accommodate the long sweeping strokes. (See Chapter 11 for tips on working with larger children.)

When massaging older children, you need to respect their need for physical privacy. This may vary, depending on the

- age of the child
- setting
- relationship of the massage giver to the child
- family and cultural preferences
- child's comfort with skin-to-skin touch
- other medical problems

You may need to drape the child with a sheet or have him or her wear a swimsuit, underwear, or shorts. Some children may feel more comfortable if you limit your massage to the back, legs (avoiding the upper thighs), feet, arms, hands, and face.

Should I continue the massage if the child is crying?

Crying is a fundamental form of communication that should be respected. Use a graded approach to introduce massage, to avoid overstimulation or disorganization. This information is applicable to children and adults. Work with the parents and the child to determine why the child is crying, and use the guidelines in Chapter 6 to find a solution.

Is it all right to focus on only one body part, such as the abdomen for the constipated child?

Yes. For example, in the case of a constipated child, often the abdomen is distended and the child is irritable. You may want to start with some gentle strokes to the back to promote relaxation, and then progress to the stomach.

What if parents do not like the idea of massage?

Not all parents (or health care professionals) are comfortable with the intimacy of massage. Respect the family's values and choose a form of tactile input that is acceptable (such as swaddling). Some people feel more comfortable with massage if it is combined with exercise such as gentle passive range of motion, stretching, or developmentally appropriate activities. Massage also can be done with a bathmit, liquid or foam soap, or a towel at bathtime. Application of body lotion or suntan lotion also is an opportunity for massage.

Which strokes should I start with?

This depends on the individual child. Often, the legs are a non-threatening place to start. Most children's legs have been handled frequently during diaper changes. Let the child's responses determine where you start. Most children tolerate massage to the legs and back well; from there move on to body parts that may be more sensitive. If a child has asymmetry in posture and sensation, begin with the more intact extremity.

How much pressure should I use?

The pressure used is gentle to accommodate small extremities but with sufficient pressure to compress the muscle belly and surrounding tissues. Relaxing your hands prior to touching the child will assist with a comforting hand placement. Each child and adult organizes tactile input differently. Some prefer slightly lighter stroking than others. Still others find a light touch to be disorganizing and prefer a firmer touch. Watch for verbal and behavioral feedback from the child, and adjust your strokes accordingly.

How should I explain massage to the child?

With an infant or severely involved child, use a calm and assuring voice. Tell the infant or child that you will be rubbing his or her arms, legs, and body. Be clear with your explanation so that the infant or child understands that he or she can let you know if he or she likes or dislikes a certain stroke. Be sure to tell the infant or child that you will stop if he or she desires. Use the parents/caregiver for interpretation of cues if you are unsure of the infant's specific cues. It is important to do this with all children, even if their cognitive or verbal level does not seem capable of being understood. Children often understand far more than they may be able to reflect in their communication.

With an older child, use a similar explanation, encouraging him or her to use words, gestures, or sign language to indicate the same preferences. This will place the child in control of the situation and relieve potential anxiety. For the older child, you may demonstrate the strokes on a doll, another child, or the parent or caregiver. The child also may want to practice by giving you a rub. Children of this age group also enjoy helping with the lotion bottle and applying lotion to themselves!

Chapter 10

Introduction

Massage is most beneficial if it is introduced when the child is in a quiet alert state. This state enables optimal interaction between child and caregiver. Refer to Chapter 4 for more information about description of states.

Massage may be viewed as a sensory integrative tactile intervention in which the child actively indicates which sensations lead to greater organization and adaptive response. The child plays an active role in the massage process and is not a passive recipient of sensory stimulation. Gestures, laughs, smiles, or verbalizations can express pleasure in response to the stroke. This provides insight into which strokes appear beneficial.

Introduce massage into a home/therapy/education program slowly; carefully evaluate the child's response to each new stroke. Introduce one set of strokes during a weekly therapy session and provide time for the caregiver to practice and observe the child's response. It is important to watch the child's cues before, during, and after the intervention. This may mean asking the parent for information about the child's response after the session.

Materials

Oils and lotions

Natural, cold-pressed nut or fruit oils/lotion should be used for massage. Cold-pressed oils are extracted from the fruit or nut and are a pure form of distillation without chemical additives. Many commercial massage oils contain additives or fragrance. Natural lotions, which are free of petroleum or chemical additives, also are readily available.

A massage using lotion may produce a slightly different friction from that of oil; choose an oil or lotion according to its contents and the child's response. These oils may be appropriate massage mediums for infants and children:

- apricot kernel
- rice bran
- safflower

- sesame
- canola
- olive

These oils are readily available at health food stores and in the natural-foods section of grocery stores. There also are bath and body shops that carry massage oils and lotions. Examine the label to determine the true content of the oil (some commercially available "almond oils" are actually mineral oil and fragrance). Natural oils may turn rancid with time; check for freshness before each use. Store the unused oil in a cool place.

Avoid products containing petroleum, such as mineral oil, as they are non-edible. During massage, children often bring a massaged hand or foot to the mouth and subsequently may ingest the oil. Use natural oils and lotions because the effects of absorption of petroleum products into the skin are unclear.

Some oils, particularly those derived from nuts such as peanut and almond oil, may produce an allergic skin reaction. *A child who is allergic to nuts most likely will be allergic to the oil.* The child's parent or physician should be consulted before the oil is applied. Because infants and young children often have not previously been exposed to nuts, it is safer to choose a vegetable oil and avoid using a nut oil until the child is older. To avoid an allergic reaction, perform a skin-patch test before using the oil. Place a small amount of oil on an area such as the wrist; wait 30 minutes to determine tolerance for the oil or lotion. If the skin is extremely sensitive, lubrication may be omitted, or strokes may be performed using a blanket, velour towel, or bath puppet. If necessary, massage also may be performed through the clothes or pajamas.

Hospitals may have specific infection-control precautions that preclude introducing oil into the nursery or pediatric environment. Consult the infection-control staff to encourage the introduction of natural oils, where possible. It has been clinically suggested that oil be avoided when the infant is placed under a radiant warmer, as this may pose the risk of a burn. A study conducted in a hospital nursery in India by Fernandez, et al. (1987) suggested that the use of corn oil, applied topically, might be beneficial in helping the preterm infant maintain body temperature and act as a source of nutrition.

Aromatherapy

Aromatherapy uses essential oils to promote the health and well-being of the mind, body, and spirit. The following information may be useful in practice. There are a number of good references available to provide background information and suggestions for use. (See the References on page 193.) Essential oils have been used for centuries for religious ceremonies, healing, and perfumes. In more recent history, aromatherapy has been used more widely in Europe than in the United States. It is becoming more popular in the U.S., particularly for use in calming and stress reduction.

Sanderson, Harrison, and Price (1991) suggested that essential oils can affect emotions and motor functions, and that smell memories can last longer than visual memories. Aromatherapy and massage may be used as a way of relieving tension and promoting relaxation. Essential oils also have invigorating and refreshing properties that can help relieve fatigue and improve concentration.

Dye (1992) discussed the sense of smell's powerful influence on the mind, as it has a direct link to the brain and central nervous system. Smell sends electrical signals through the olfactory bulb into the limbic system, which also is known as the emotional center of the brain. Smell has a profound effect on long-term and short-term memory as well as emotions. Smell can provide a powerful, conditioned response that may be used therapeutically with children and adults. If a child associates a certain scent with relaxation, that scent may be used during stressful situations or transitions during the day. The authors have used lavender with their children as a method of reducing stress and helping these children cope with transition times such as getting ready for bed. In clinical practice, the authors noted that lavender was helpful in relieving stress in an adolescent girl diagnosed with autism. Her mother continues to use lavender as a method of self-calming and decreasing anxiety.

Essential oils are extracted by steam distillation or direct expression from aromatic plants. These oils may be purchased at health food stores, some grocery stores, or through aromatherapists and their suppliers. A few drops of essential oil are mixed with vegetable carrier oils for use in massage. Essential oils are flammable and highly concentrated. They are typically sold in small, dark glass vials to provide protection from sunlight. They should be stored in a cool, dry area. Essential oils *should not* be placed directly on the skin, as they may potentially burn the skin due to their extreme concentration. The American Cancer Society's website (1997) noted that essential oils should not be taken internally because they can be poisonous, and that prolonged exposure to essential oils can cause allergic reactions. *Do not use essential oils near or in the eyes.*

Essential oils commonly used with children and their uses: (IAIM, 1997; Higley & Higley, 1998)

- Blue chamomile—Calms and soothes
- Eucalyptus and Peppermint—Helps relieve respiratory congestion
- Geranium—Acts as a mild sedative and anti-depressant
- Lavender—Acts as a mild sedative and helps regulate sleep patterns
- Tangerine—Helps with colic and stomach aches
- Ylang-Ylang—Calms and relaxes
- Eucalyptus—Promotes deeper respiration
- Peppermint—Promotes alertness

These oils are used in a carrier lotion, added to the water in a child's bath, or placed on a cotton ball near the child. They are never used directly on the skin.

There appear to be wide variations in recommended uses and contraindications for essential oils. Some researchers suggest that some essential oils are considered toxic (Dye, 1992; Sanderson, Harrison, & Price, 1991). Research the available information or consult an aromatherapist before using any oil. Certain oils are contraindicated for certain conditions, such as pregnancy and asthma; thus, the massage giver and recipient must be aware of potential toxicity.

Sanderson, Harrison, and Price (1991) discussed contraindications and considerations for use of essential oils with massage, including working with people with asthma, epilepsy, or cancer. They suggested that the number of drops of essential oil used for children should be half of that recommended for adults. Aromatherapy offers an additional sensory input that may be therapeutic when combined with massage. It also decreases stress and promotes feelings of wellness. The growing popularity of aromatherapy supports the powerful sensation of smell (Dye, 1992; Price & Parr, 1996; Sanderson, Harrison, & Price, 1991).

Although research has not validated the use of aromatherapy, there have been some emerging studies exploring the effectiveness of using lavender and rosemary (Buckle, 1993; Diego et. al, in press). Clinically, success, in the form of decreasing stress and promoting relaxation is achieved while using specific essential oils.

Preparation

- Warm the carrier (vegetable, fruit or nut) oil prior to massage by placing the bottle in heated water or rubbing it in your hands. Do not microwave it as there may be hot pockets that can burn.

- Diapers, a blanket, towels, and positioning equipment should be readily available.

- Trim fingernails and remove jewelry to provide smooth input during strokes, and to prevent scratching.

- Have small toys available for manipulative play as needed.

- Musical toys or mirrors, placed underneath the child where he or she can see them, can be particularly nice during massage in prone.

Environment

Warmth

- The environment should be warm and comfortable for the child, as the child will be undressed during the massage.

- A soft and warm surface such as a thermal blanket or sheepskin is excellent for massage.

- Clean towels heated in a clothes dryer will assure that the child is lying on a warm surface.

- Use additional blankets to drape body parts not being massaged, or leave the child partly clothed.

- The massage giver's hands should be warm.

Auditory

Decrease excessive noise as much as possible. In a clinic environment, you may need to find an enclosed room where distraction will be minimal.

Relaxation music may be used if it appears to aid in the child's organization. Some selections include

- "Lullaby Magic" (Bartels)
- "Lullabies from Around the World," "Slumberland," "Sweet Baby Dreams" (Bergman)
- "Lullabies and Sweet Dreams" (Halpern)
- "Spectrum Suite" (Steven Halpern, 1979 Halpern Sounds)
- "Winter into Spring," "December," "Autumn" (George Winston December, 1982 Windham Hill Records)
- Pachelbel: Canon in D major and other baroque selections (Great Performances Great Baroque Favorites, 1983 ,CBS, Inc.)
- Baby Go to Sleep
- The Fairy Ring (Mike Rowland, 1990, Enso Records)
- Mozart Effect Music for Children (Don Campbell, 1997, The Children's Group, Inc.)

A narrated story also may prove calming to some children. Sounds of nature, such as waves, forests, rain, or intrauterine sounds, also can provide relaxation. Commercially available sound machines now simulate heartbeats, streams, fountains, and ocean sounds. These may prove useful for calming the child with irritability.

The lethargic child may benefit from marches and other upbeat music. Older children may enjoy music in which they can participate, such as

- "Singable Songs for the Very Young" (Raffi)
- Discovery Toys: "Sounds like Fun"
- Disney songs
- Wee Sing songs
- Tim Noah songs

Music therapists are excellent resources for music choices in therapy/educational programs. It is important also to consider the cultural issues behind music selection. Some music classified as *new age* may feel uncomfortable to some families. Therefore, it is very important to include family and caregivers in the selection of music for massage.

Lighting

The fluorescent lighting common in clinics and hospitals emits a high-frequency flickering that is irritating to some children. Rooms with dim incandescent lights or natural sunlight may be a relaxing change and may enhance the child's ability to focus.

Relaxation

Relax before initiating the massage—adult stress often is communicated to children. Progressive muscle relaxation, gentle stretching, deep breathing, and imagery are useful relaxation techniques. Choose massage positions that are comfortable for you and promote healthy body alignment. Parents, caregivers, and interventionists also should treat themselves to a professional massage or a simple back rub from a friend.

Chapter 11

General Positioning Principles

Introduction

Positioning during massage should take into account the child's age, muscle tone, medical condition, postural responses to gravity, reflex activity, vision/hearing, and level of interaction. Consult the child's physical or occupational therapist to get information about creative, functional alternatives for positioning. Good positioning will help ensure a successful massage experience.

Supine and Prone

The most common positions for pediatric massage are the **supine** (back lying) position and the **prone** (stomach lying) position.

The Supine Position

This is the preferred position for massage, as it gives the best opportunity for eye contact and interaction. This position also gives the interventionist the best clues about the child's reaction to the input. The caregiver should sit comfortably, with the back supported. The child may be positioned on a pillow or wedge in front of the massage-giver. If sitting on the floor is difficult for the caregiver, the child could be placed on an elevated surface such as a bed or table so that the adult may be seated in a chair or standing. The very small infant can be in a supine tuck on the caregiver's lap. This may help promote a sense of midline orientation for him or her.

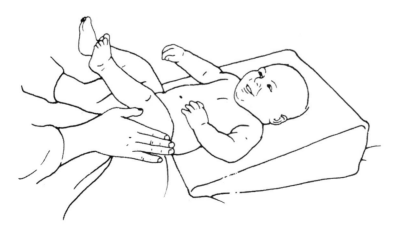

The desired elements of the supine position for massage include

- head in midline with slight chin tuck and cervical elongation

- shoulders forward (avoid shoulder elevation) and in neutral depression

- arms in approximately 45° to 90° of shoulder-forward flexion, elbows slightly flexed, and neutral alignment of the forearm

- hips slightly flexed

- legs in neutral position. Avoid excessive scissoring (adduction/internal rotation) or frogged position (extreme abduction/external rotation). A wedge or towel roll may be placed between the legs to prevent scissoring of the legs. Additionally, pillows or beanbags may help prevent external rotation and abduction (frogged position).

The Prone Position

To massage a child in prone, position the child over your lap with the shoulders forward, or use a wedge, roll, or half roll to provide support for the child.

The desired elements of this position for massage include

- head in midline

- shoulders and arms forward

- legs in neutral positioning to prevent excessive scissoring or extreme abduction. A wedge or bolster may be used to prevent scissoring or a frogged position.

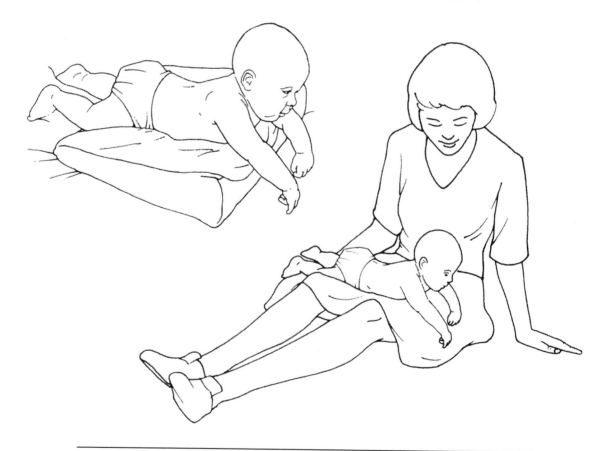

Other positions

Many alternative positions, such as **sidelying, sitting, prone suspension** (the football hold), and **at the shoulder,** are available for special circumstances. These positions may be preferred for

- the large child

- the child with strong asymmetry

- the child with extreme extensor or flexor posturing

- the child with muscle tone that cannot be adequately controlled in prone or supine

- the mobile child

- the child who wishes to remain close to the parent or caretaker

- the child with medical equipment (e.g., a G-tube, tracheostomy, ventilator)

- the child with gastro-esophageal reflux

Sidelying

The influence of extensor posturing in supine and flexor posturing in prone may make positioning difficult. This could be further complicated by excessive hypertonicity or hypotonicity, which may inhibit antigravity control and mobility. Sidelying may be a useful alternative for the child whose tone cannot be controlled adequately in supine or prone.

Wedges, bolsters, or towels may be used to position the child comfortably in sidelying. For larger children, use an elevated surface such as a bed or table and pillows to provide proper positioning. A sidelyer also may be used for the very large child.

The desired elements of the sidelying position for massage include

- slight chin tuck with cervical elongation

- neutral position of the trunk without excessive flexion or extension

- arms forward at approximately 90°

- legs in flexion or with a dissociated position (hip and knee flexion on the leg, and hip and knee extension on the other). This will help reduce increased extension. Use pillows and rolls to achieve this position.

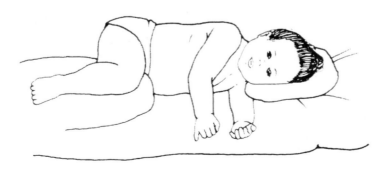

Sitting

This position is useful in a variety of situations. Some children feel uncomfortable or threatened in supine. Sitting may enable more freedom to play and also is helpful for the mobile child. In addition, you also can be highly interactive with the child in sitting, as in supine. For example, you can incorporate hand-play games as a part of the massage.

At first, sitting may be the only position you can use with the child. Some strokes can be introduced at bath time, using the water or soft-soap as a medium.

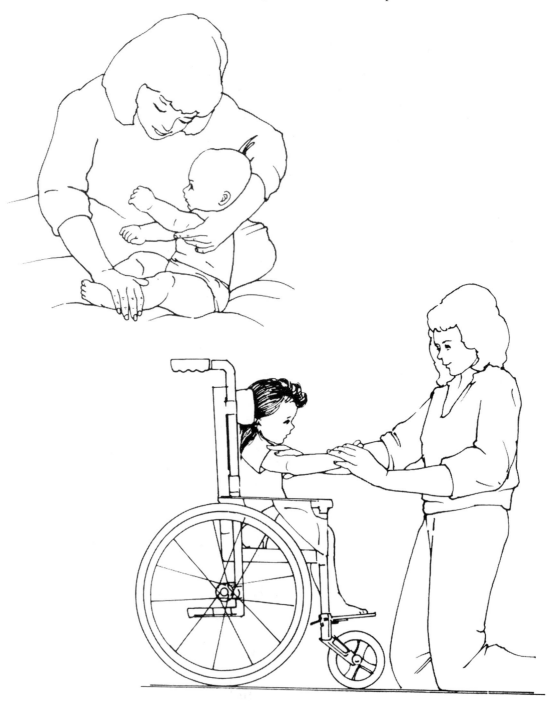

Prone Suspension—the Football Hold

Prone suspension is one way to provide abdominal massage. Gravity in combination with the child's body weight over the caretaker's hand gives slight pressure into the abdomen area. This may be combined with slight forward and backward movement to offer calming vestibular input. Parents often use this technique for calming young infants.

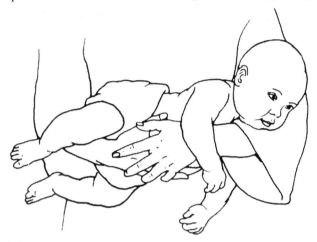

At the Shoulder

Some children need the comfort of being held, before massage can begin. Being massaged at the shoulder can provide relaxation, too. Sometimes, after a series of strokes to the back, the child will allow some stroking in either prone or supine. The Kangaroo Care Method supports the important benefits of ventral-to-ventral contact encouraged by this position (Anderson, 1991).

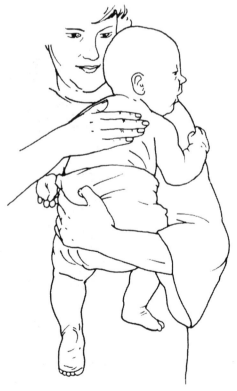

Positioning Devices

The following positioning devices also may be used to achieve appropriate positioning during massage:

- the child's seating system

- a flexistander

- a beanbag chair

- a prone stander

- dynamic pieces of equipment (e.g., hammock, platform swing)

- bath chair

- car seat

- infant seat

- a supportive chair

Summary

Try to base the massage position on principles of therapeutic handling, positioning, and the child's comfort. At times, you may need to choose between an optimum position and a position that enables greater eye contact and interaction. At this point, consider the specific therapeutic/educational goals desired for the child. Positioning is meant to provide comfort and support so that the child may receive maximal benefits from the massage.

Chapter 12

Massage Strokes

Introduction

The following massage strokes have been adapted from the work of Vimala Schneider McClure to accommodate the specific needs of special children (McClure, 1989). Based on concepts of neurodevelopmental theory, sensory integrative theory, and functional biomechanics, these strokes have been modified to accommodate infants/children with varying diagnoses, skills, and needs. It is important to note that no massage will be identical, as children present with such varied sensory, motor, communication, social, emotional, and behavioral issues. The interventionist must be flexible in assessing the child's strengths and needs first, and developing a massage program in conjunction with parents, caregivers, and the multidisciplinary team.

These strokes, which are a combination of Indian and Swedish massage techniques, balance excitatory and inhibitory sensory input to the nervous system. The strokes also take into account the issues of postural control, sensory integration, and positioning needs. Therapeutic handling principles have been incorporated to produce optimal results for the massage giver and the child.

Many texts describe massage strokes for children; a number of them are listed in the bibliography. It is recommended that you explore the various resources—and use your own creativity—in designing a massage program that meets the unique characteristics of the specific child and family.

When planning the program, carefully examine the family's priorities and the individual's treatment/educational plan. Take into account such issues as

- social interaction,

- muscle tone,

- language/communication,

- visual/auditory skill,

- range of motion,

- sensitivity to sensory stimulation,

- active movement, and

- family preferences.

Choose the strokes that will accomplish the specific goals for each child.

The most important cues will be the child's response and communication of which strokes bring pleasure. Be sure to follow the child's lead and actively respond to the nonverbal and verbal requests. Here is one suggested sequence of strokes. Depending on the circumstances, you may prefer to devise your own. The order of presentation depends on many of the aforementioned factors. Depending on age and developmental skill, the child may prefer a seated massage as opposed to prone or supine.

Lower Extremities

1. Indian Milking—Away From the Heart
2. Wringing
3. Thumb Press
4. Squeeze Each Toe
5. Stroke Top of Foot
6. Circles Around the Ankles
7. Swedish Milking—Toward the Heart
8. Rolling

Abdomen

1. Gentle Pressure on the Abdomen
2. Paddle Wheel
3. Paddle Wheel With Legs Lifted
4. Sun Moon
5. I Love You
6. Gentle Pressure on the Abdomen

Chest

1. Heart
2. Criss-Cross
3. Shoulder to Toes

Upper Extremities

1. Symmetrical Starting Stroke
2. Indian Milking—Away From the Heart
3. Wringing
4. Thumb Press in Palm
5. Small Circles in Palm
6. Squeeze Each Finger
7. Stroke Top of Hand
8. Circles Around the Wrist
9. Swedish Milking—Toward the Heart
10. Rolling

Back

1. Swooping to the Bottom
2. Swooping to the Ankles
3. Back and Forth
4. Small Circles All Over the Back
5. Combing

Face

1. Forehead to Mouth
2. Eyebrows to Mouth
3. Nose to Mouth
4. Pressure Toward the Mouth
5. Finishing Stroke for the Face

Making Contact

If the child is comfortable in supine, place your relaxed hands gently around the child's hips and provide some slight rocking. Talk to the child; tell the child that you will be touching the legs. Wait for cues for engagement (e.g., eye contact, smiling, verbal cues), as this is an interactive experience.

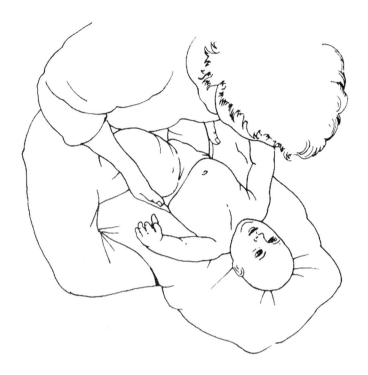

To provide a more organizing sensation throughout the massage, try to maintain **one stable point of contact**—one hand should always be touching the body, even during the transition between strokes. Those who have had a massage in which the hands are on and off in an erratic manner can attest to the disorganization of this sensory input. It also is important that your hands be warm and relaxed. Hands should make contact and be taken off gently and slowly to avoid a startle.

Lower Extremities

Clinical experience suggests that beginning with the legs is the most successful. Most infants and children are best able to accept initial touch either to the legs or the back, as opposed to other body parts. Caregivers appear to be more comfortable touching and playing with their children's legs (i.e., changing diapers or playing "bicycle").

All the strokes in the leg series are completed on one leg before beginning on the other. This enables you to compare the significant difference in skin coloration and temperature between the massaged and the unmassaged leg. Many children may experience poor circulation in their lower extremities due to limited movement, thus this is a welcome benefit.

If a child is able to tolerate stimulation to the foot without adverse effect in tone or behavior, the strokes for the legs can proceed to the toes. If the child cannot tolerate input to the feet, perhaps in subsequent massages you may slowly work up to incorporating the feet. For simplicity, the following instructions describe the movement as toward the ankle.

If the child is more sensitive on one side or presents with hemiplegia, begin with the leg that has the most intact sensation and movement. This enables the child to accurately interpret the tactile information.

1. Indian Milking—Away From the Heart

Apply firm but gentle pressure, stroking from hip to ankle, alternating your hand between the inner (medial) and outer (lateral) aspects of the lower extremity.

Stroke primarily with the palm of your hand to assure a more even tactile input. Different thumb positions produce different sensations. Experiment with your thumbs held close to your index fingers and with them spread around the extremity. Use the thumb position that is most comfortable for you and the child. For the premature infant, use the web space between your thumb and index finger. The input should be directed to cover the circumference of the entire extremity.

The stroke

1. Support the leg at the inside ankle with one hand. Stroke the leg from the outer border of the thigh to the ankle with your other hand.

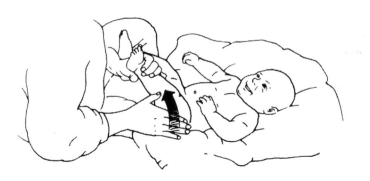

2. Alternate hands. Stroke from the inner thigh to the ankle.

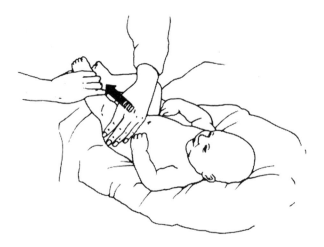

3. Continue to alternate inside and outside strokes, moving from the hip to the ankle.

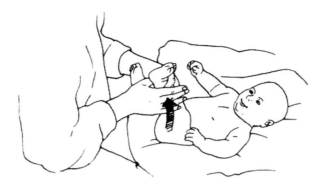

Clinical Implications—This stroke goes with the pattern of hair growth, and thus, tends to produce inhibition or relaxation. It often is useful for children with increased muscle tone as the pressure is very rhythmical and even. Most children enjoy this stroke, as it produces a pleasurable response. In the Indian culture, this stroke is believed to remove stress or negative energy (McClure, 1989).

Use this stroke therapeutically to elongate the hamstring and adductor musculature. Stroking the legs promotes visual attention to the feet, assisting in visual convergence and downward visual gaze. Because this stroke fosters an increased visual recognition of the legs, it also promotes body awareness. This stroke is an excellent preparation for lower-extremity weight bearing. The distal direction of the stroke offers the opportunity for traction that may activate the hip musculature.

2. Wringing

This is a gentle squeeze-and-twist motion from the hip to the ankle.

The stroke

1. Wrap your hands around the leg at the thigh.

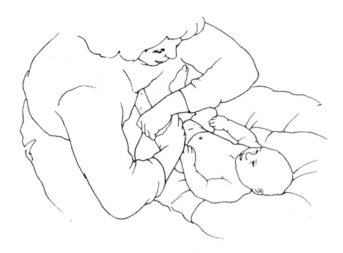

2. Gently wring the leg in both directions by twisting your hands together and then apart. Simultaneously glide your hands toward the ankle.

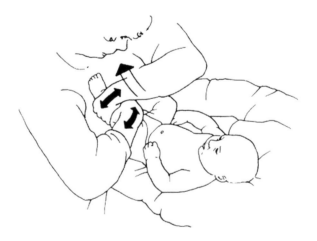

3. As your hands come to the ankle, bring one hand back to the hip, and follow with the other hand. This assures consistent tactile contact.

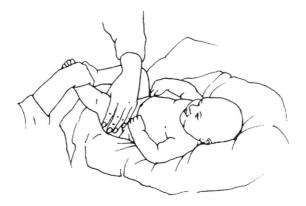

4. Repeat.

Clinical Implications—This stroke produces a cross-fiber friction motion as it gently compresses muscle and connective tissue against bone. The stroke assists in mobilizing and elongating the soft tissues of the hamstring, quadriceps, and gastrocnemius. It also may help soften adhesions and tightness in musculature, often resulting in a softer and more supple muscle belly. It may be a useful stroke to prepare for lower-extremity weight bearing. Wringing tends to be more excitatory, which makes some children uncomfortable. Use adequate lubrication during this stroke.

3. Thumb Press

This stroke provides maintained pressure on the bottom of the foot.

In some infant massage texts, there is brisk stroking to the bottom of the feet. This may be too over-stimulating for the majority of children with special needs. It is modified to produce a calming, deep pressure to the bottom of the foot.

Many children and adults with intact neurological functioning are particularly sensitive to being touched on their feet. Sensitivity often seems to be heightened in children with neurological impairment. If the massage is to be pleasurable, you must respect this.

The stroke

1. Give firm pressure to the bottom of the foot for at least 3 to 5 seconds. Use either your thumb or the padded area of your palm under your thumb (the *thenar eminence*).

2. Move your hand slowly and only a small distance to apply pressure to adjacent areas (as in step 1).

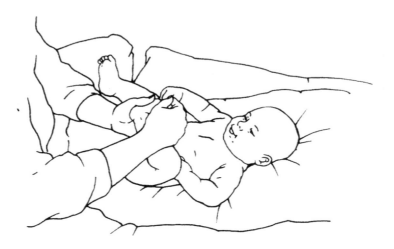

If the child cannot tolerate the stimulation caused by the moving pressure, use your entire palm to apply steady pressure to the entire bottom of the foot.

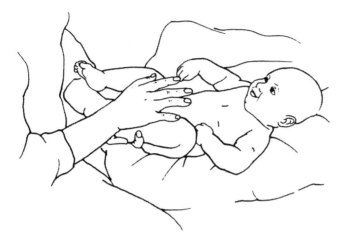

Clinical Implications—It is important that the child receive pleasurable and therapeutic input to the feet for purposes of weight bearing. Many children have had unpleasant sensory stimuli such as multiple heel sticks and have extreme sensitivity in their feet. This stroke provides a method of helping reduce that sensitivity and enabling the child to accept more tactile input to the feet. Observe the child's response and carefully grade the input to the feet. Touch to the feet may cause increased extensor tone or discomfort in some children. To prevent this increase in tone and associated toe curling, hold the foot with the toes in slight extension and the ankle in approximately 90 degrees of dorsiflexion, if range of motion is available.

4. Squeeze Each Toe

This is a gentle rolling and squeezing of each toe.

Many children are particularly sensitive to touch at their toes. Proceed slowly while monitoring the child's response to the input. This is a good time to introduce language games such as "This Little Piggy" or counting games.

The stroke

1. Gently grasp the base of the large toe (on the top and bottom surface) between your thumb and index finger.

2. Slide your fingers from the base to the tip of the toe, using a gentle rolling, squeezing motion.

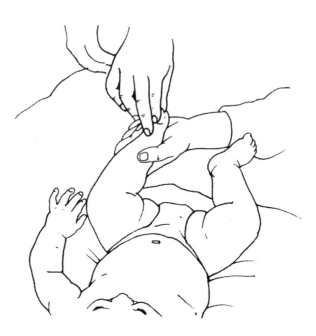

3. Repeat this motion with each toe, in order.

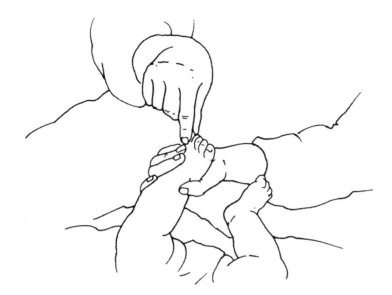

Clinical Implications—This stroke also offers the opportunity to visually regard the feet and legs. Children may spontaneously reach for their feet, promoting forward reach and trunk flexion. This reach also may serve to elongate the hamstring musculature. If the child cannot tolerate this input to the individual toes or has very lax ligaments, gently but firmly cup all the toes simultaneously between the pads of your fingers and your palm. If child with tight toe flexion can tolerate the cupping, you also may provide a gentle stretch to the toes and underlying fascia.

5. Stroke Top of Foot

This is a stroking motion toward the heart.

The stroke

1. Stabilize the foot with one hand by cupping it around the heel.

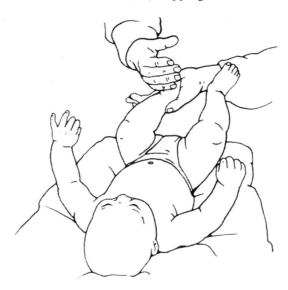

2. Stroke the top of the foot from the toes to the front of the lower leg.

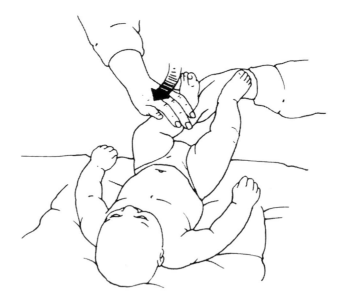

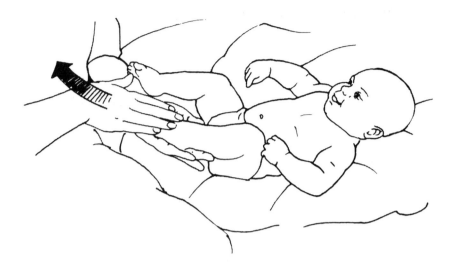

3. Repeat.

If the ankle is tight into dorsiflexion/eversion, change the direction of the stroke so that it proceeds from the front of the lower leg to the toes. (This pattern of tightness often is present in preterm infants.)

Clinical Implications—This stroke may be used to promote isolated dorsiflexion of the ankle. It is important to get the calcaneous (*heel bone*) in neutral alignment while performing this stroke, as many children present with either inversion or eversion. Consult the child's physical therapist for specific concerns related to structural issues of the feet.

6. Circle Around the Ankles

This is a continuous stroke completely encircling the bony area (the *malleoli*) of the ankles.

The stroke

1. Stabilize the foot in neutral alignment with both hands, supporting the heel with your fingers.

2. Move your thumbs simultaneously in a circle around the ankles.

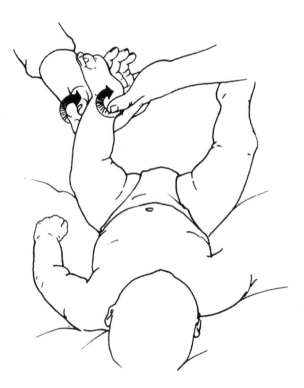

Clinical Implications—The skin around the malleoli often is fragile in some children who are very thin. This presents skin-breakdown issues with children requiring orthotics. This stroke may serve to improve circulation to that area and assist with prevention of breakdown. This stroke is sometimes difficult to coordinate. It may be easier to use the index and middle fingers of one hand to perform the circular motion while you stabilize the foot with the other hand. Use the technique most comfortable for you.

7. Swedish Milking—Toward the Heart

Apply firm but gentle pressure, moving from ankle to hip followed by a lighter stroke back toward the foot. Hands alternate between the outer (lateral) and inner (medial) surfaces of the extremity.

The stroke

1. Support the leg with one hand at the inside ankle. Use the other hand to stroke firmly from the ankle to the hip on the outside surface of the leg.

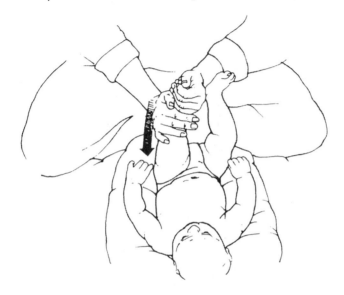

2. Stroke around the hip, without breaking contact.

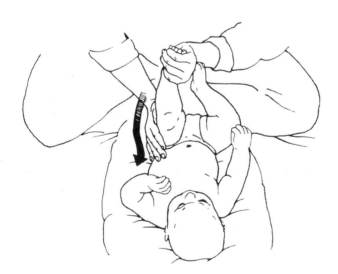

3. Stroke back toward the ankle, using your finger pads and a lighter pressure.

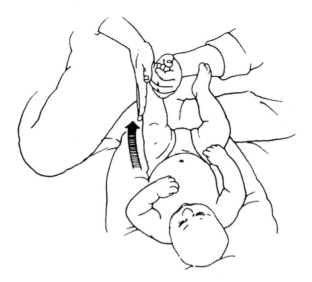

4. Switch hands by supporting the leg at the outside ankle. Use your other hand to stroke firmly from the inner ankle to the inner thigh.

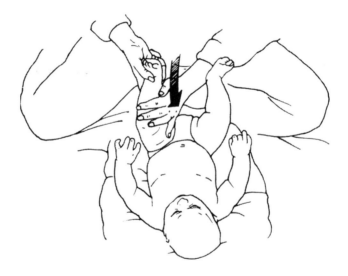

5. Stroke back toward the ankle, using your finger pads and a lighter pressure.

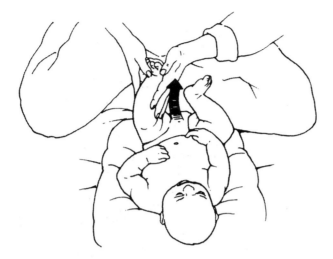

6. Repeat the stroke, alternating your hands.

Clinical Implications—This stroke may be used as Indian Milking to elongate the hamstring and adductor musculature with proper alignment. Combine range of motion with this stroke as long as it doesn't interfere with the child's enjoyment. As muscle tissue becomes more supple, range of motion often is easier to obtain. Swedish massage strokes tend to be more excitatory because there is movement against the pattern of hair growth, as well as a mechanical pumping of blood back to the heart, aiding venous return. Monitor the child's behavior to determine whether the stroke is well-tolerated. This stoke offers a balance of excitation and inhibition, but may be too stimulating for some children. If so, use Indian Milking instead. Sometimes, it is fun to use sounds or rhythmical music in conjunction with these strokes.

8. Rolling

This is a gentle rolling finishing stroke of the leg, moving from hip to ankle.

The stroke

1. Place the flat part of your palms on the inner and outer surfaces of the upper thigh.

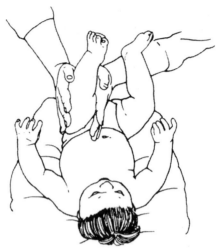

2. Gently alternate your hands to produce a rolling motion (like rolling dough). Simultaneously glide your hands toward the foot while rolling.

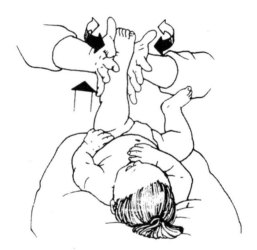

3. Pause a moment when your hands have reached the ankle to enable the child to accommodate the input before repeating the stroke.

4. Maintain one hand at the ankle and reposition the other hand at the hip, ensuring continual contact.

5. Repeat.

Clinical Implications—Most children enjoy this stroke which often initiates a playful and communicative interaction. This is an ideal time to wait between strokes for a verbal or nonverbal indication that the child wants more. One child with visual impairment indicated the desire for more by pushing both feet up in the air. Others may verbalize or sign more. This is an opportune time to encourage that communication.

If the child cannot handle this input, gently pat the leg from hip to ankle as a finishing stroke. If there is a potential for hip subluxation, you may choose gentle hand placement around the hip to finish the series of lower-extremity strokes. Also, if the child is large, roll the leg from the ankle to the knee first, then the knee to the foot. This will prevent the possibility of lateral movement at the knee.

Abdomen

Many children with special needs have difficulty maintaining a regular pattern of elimination. Caregivers often are frustrated with typical remedies such as prune juice, laxatives, or suppositories. Abdominal massage offers a natural alternative that gently encourages elimination. Some bowel management protocols for children with spina bifida include massage strokes to the abdomen. It also is important to note that children with diagnosed gastrointestinal disorders may be uncomfortable with massage to their abdomen.

The strokes to the abdomen generally move from the child's right to left (your left to right). This is the direction of movement of fecal matter through the large intestine.

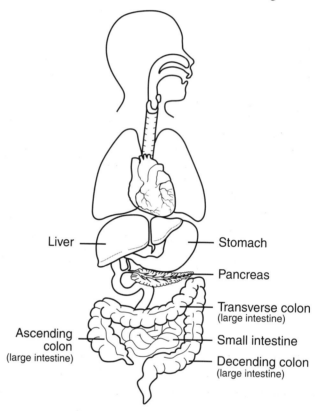

Liver

Stomach

Pancreas

Transverse colon
(large intestine)

Ascending
colon
(large intestine)

Small intestine

Decending colon
(large intestine)

The abdomen should not be massaged immediately after a feeding. To avoid hicupping, spitting up, vomiting, or discomfort, wait at least 30 to 45 minutes after the child has eaten before beginning the stomach massage. You will need to slightly lower the child's diaper or at least open it, in order to effectively massage the abdomen. This must be done at the discretion of the family and the child. For the strokes to be most effective and comfortable, concentrate stroking on the area between the lowest rib and the pubic bone.

Firm, yet gentle, pressure to the stomach can produce overall relaxation. It is commonly combined with a gentle touch to the head to soothe infants in intensive care units. Be aware that many infants and children are very sensitive, especially to light touch in this area. Proceed slowly and gradually if the child gives an indication of sensitivity.

1. Gentle Pressure on the Abdomen

This stroke is a hand placement with gentle pressure to the abdomen.

This is a nice way to begin the abdominal massage. It enables the child to organize and integrate the tactile input to the stomach before proceeding to the stroking. Repeat at the end of the abdominal massage as a finishing stroke.

The stroke

1. Place your relaxed hand on the abdomen at the level of the navel.

2. Maintain this point of contact for a brief time and watch for cues of organization or engagement.

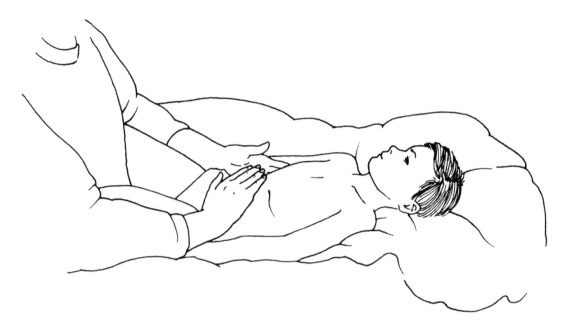

Clinical Implications—This initially may be the only stroke sensitive children can tolerate without discomfort. With continued massage, most children are able to transition to other abdominal massage strokes. This gentle hand placement also may be used between a series of strokes to other body parts to bring the child back to midline orientation.

2. Paddle Wheel

This stroke is a hand-over-hand movement down the center of the abdomen.

Most children tolerate this stroke well, as it tends to be soothing.

The stroke

1. Place one hand in the center of the child's abdomen, below the rib cage.

2. Glide the hand down toward the groin area.

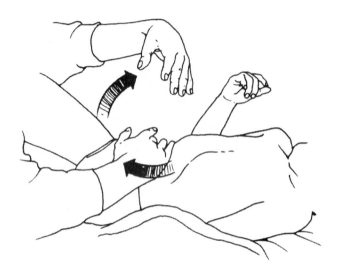

3. Repeat with the other hand, making a paddling motion.

4. Continue alternating hands. Make sure one hand is always in contact with the stomach.

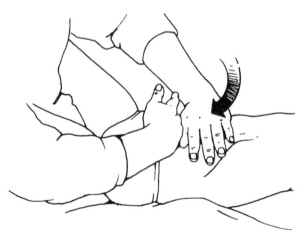

Clinical Implications—For a small baby, use only the pads of two or three fingers.

3. Paddle Wheel With Legs Lifted

Similar to the Paddle Wheel, but one hand strokes while the other hand positions the hips with greater flexion.

The stroke

1. Hold both legs with one hand at the ankle. Lift legs, flexing hips to approximately 90°.

2. Stroke with the other hand as in the Paddle Wheel.

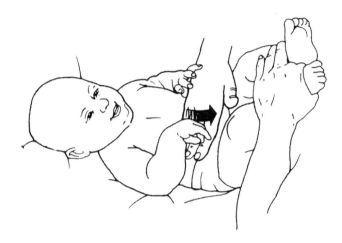

Clinical Implications—This stroke massages the stomach more deeply. This stroke may be used to provide sensory input to the abdomen before proceeding to the clockwise strokes.

4. Sun Moon

In this stroke, both hands move in a clockwise direction.

Your left hand will always be in contact with the skin. The right hand must lift off the surface at times in order to move over your left hand. Practice on a doll until you can perform the stroke smoothly and rhythmically. This may prove to be a challenge of bilateral coordination, yet with practice, it is a nice addition to the series of abdominal massage strokes.

The stroke

1. Move your left hand (the *sun*) in a continuous clockwise circle.

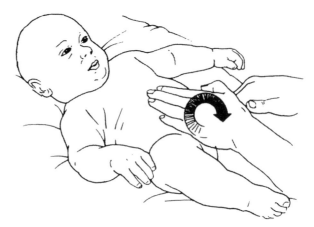

2. Imagine a clock face on the child's stomach. When your left hand reaches 6 o'clock, your right hand (the *moon*) will move in a semicircle from your left (9 o'clock) to your right (3 o'clock).

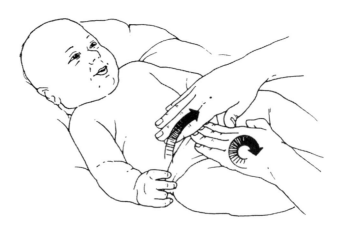

3. Lift your right hand over your left, to return to the 9 o'clock position.

4. Repeat in a continuous motion.

Clinical Implications—This stroke emphasizes movement of material through the large intestine as it moves in a clockwise manner. Many parents and clinicians have found this stroke to be helpful for relieving gas and constipation. Another alternative is to simply move one hand in a clockwise circle on the abdomen. Increase the pressure while moving from the 9 o'clock to the 3 o'clock position.

5. I Love You

This is a three-part stroke that generally follows the path of the large intestine.

Children especially enjoy this stroke when it is accompanied by the words *I love you.*

Place your nondominant hand on the child's hip to maintain a point of contact and use your dominant hand to perform the strokes. Or, switch hands for each of the three parts, making sure that one hand is always in contact with the child.

The stroke

1. Starting well below the rib cage on the child's left side (your right), move your hand straight down, as if forming the letter *I.*

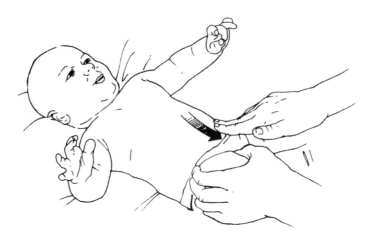

2. Place your hand on the child's right side (your left) well below the ribs. Glide your hand across to the child's left side (your right) and then downward. This forms a rotated *L.*

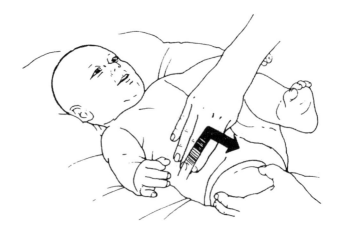

3. Place your hand near the child's right hip (your left). Move up, across the abdomen, and down near the child's left hip (your right) in the pattern of an upside-down *U*.

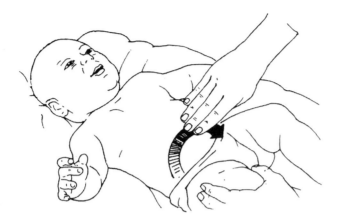

Clinical Implications—This stroke facilitates movement of matter through the large intestine.

- The *I* stroke moves in the direction of the *descending colon.*

- The *love* stroke moves in the direction of the transverse and descending colon.

- The *you* stroke moves in the direction of the ascending, transverse, and descending colon.

This stroke often is very helpful for relief of gas and constipation.

6. Gentle Pressure on the Abdomen

This stroke is a hand placement with gentle pressure to the abdomen.

This is a nice way to begin the abdominal massage. It enables the child to organize and integrate the tactile input to the stomach before proceeding to the stroking. Repeat at the end of the abdominal massage as a finishing stroke.

The stroke

1. Place your relaxed hand on the abdomen at the level of the navel.

2. Maintain this point of contact for a brief time and watch for cues of organization or engagement.

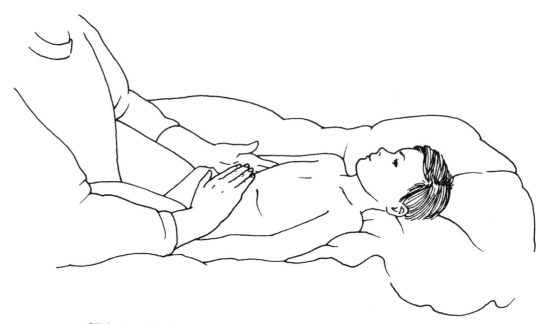

Clinical Implications—This initially may be the only stroke sensitive children can tolerate without discomfort. With continued massage, most children are able to transition to other abdominal massage strokes. This gentle hand placement also may be used between a series of strokes to other body parts to bring the child back to midline orientation.

Chest

The chest and shoulders are particularly sensitive in typically developing infants and those with special needs. At first, the child may be able to accept only the placement of your hands at the center of the chest. Some children seem initially toprefer a gentle clapping on the chest as opposed to stroking.

Some therapists have suggested that the chest massage may be a soothing preparation and follow-up to chest percussion treatment. You also may work on elongating the pectoral and intercostal musculature in coordination with the child's treatment plan. During and after the chest massage, children often have deeper respiration and more efficient phonation/vocalization. There often is more volume with greater length of vocalization.

1. Heart

In this stroke, the hands glide out from midline, down, and back up toward the center.

The stroke

1. Place your hands at the midline of the child's chest, below the clavicle.

2. Glide the hands out to the sides.

3. Slide the hands downward along the sides of the chest to the lower border of the rib cage.

4. Move the hands together and back to the starting point.

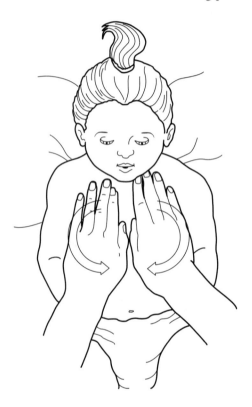

Clinical Implications—Think of this stroke as outlining a heart shape on the child's chest, or tracing the child's lungs. If indicated, work on elongating the pectoral muscles during this stroke. It also is important to emphasize *shaping* the child's rib cage, as many children present with flaring of the rib cage. This flaring may occur due to inactivity of the oblique abdominals and limited antigravity movement. While finishing this stroke, emphasize movement that brings the rib cage toward proper alignment. It is important to coordinate downward pressure on the chest with exhalation.

2. Criss-Cross

In this stroke, alternating hands move in diagonals from the hip to the opposite shoulder.

This stroke can be very rhythmical and relaxing. Be sure to maintain even pressure during this stroke. Children who are sensitive to tactile input at the chest often prefer the Heart stroke to this stroke.

The stroke

1. Place your hands at the child's hips.

2. Slide your left hand diagonally from the child's right hip up to the child's opposite shoulder.

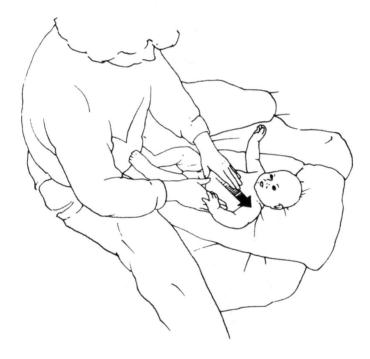

3. Without lifting your left hand, slide it back down to the starting point.

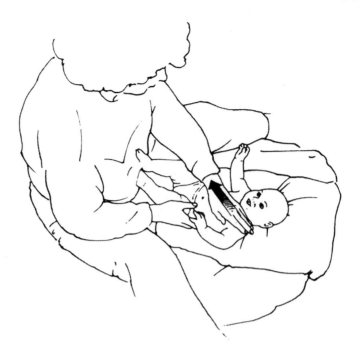

4. Slide your right hand from the child's left hip to the opposite shoulder.

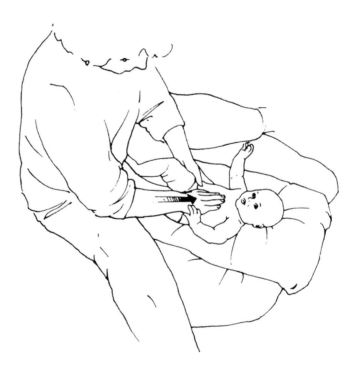

5. Without lifting your right hand, slide it back down to the starting point.

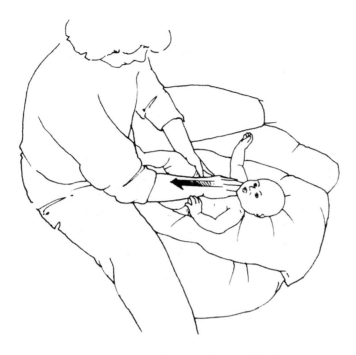

6. Repeat. This will make an *X* pattern on the child's chest.

Clinical Implications—This stroke emphasizes pectoral elongation and shoulder depression. For children with tightness in the shoulder girdle and rib cage, this stroke offers increased mobility and improved respiration. You also may combine this stroke with diagonal movement of the arm, and proceed up the arm. This provides excellent mobility to the shoulder girdle. If the child responds adversely to touch at the top of the shoulder, stroke only up to the chest. Gradually lengthen the stroke to include the shoulder.

3. Shoulder to Toes

This is a finishing stroke down the sides of the trunk from the shoulder to the toes.

The stroke

1. Place your hands at the child's shoulders.

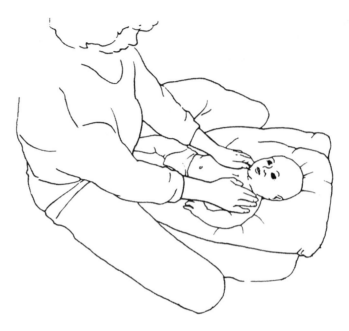

2. Glide the hands downward in unison, gently following the contours of the child's trunk, hips, and legs. Continue to the feet if the stroke does not cause adverse reaction or an abnormal foot position.

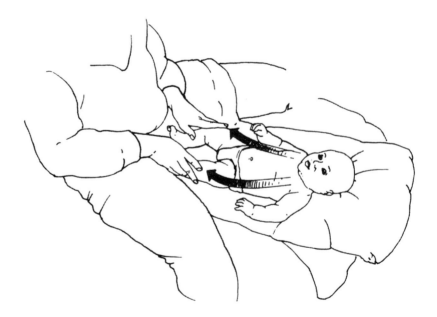

3. Bring one hand back up to the shoulder while the other hand maintains contact at the ankle or the foot.

4. Bring the other hand up to the shoulder.

5. Repeat.

Clinical Implications—This stroke may enhance body scheme by providing a sense of connection between the shoulders, chest, abdomen, legs, and feet. It is fun to sing a song such as "Head, shoulders, knees, and toes" with this stroke to emphasize body concept.

Upper Extremities

The shoulder girdle often is a vulnerable area for the child who has neuromotor impairment. Introduce upper-extremity strokes only after successfully massaging less sensitive body parts such as the back or the legs. It usually is best to massage the extremity with the most intact sensation, tone, and movement first, and then proceed to the more involved extremity. As with the legs, massage one arm completely before beginning the other.

Consider the child's developmental level when you massage the arms. If a young infant is in a pattern of physiological flexion, massage with the arms in that position—don't try to fully extend them. For an older child, you may begin the massage if the arms are pulled tightly into flexion; use therapy techniques to gently extend them, with the forearm in neutral or slight in supination. This will enable the child to experience the full input of the long, sweeping strokes.

The strokes for the upper extremities provide an excellent preparation for introduction of other therapy techniques. After elongation and relaxation of the soft tissues have occurred, it is an opportune time to work on weight bearing, active reach, grasp, and functional play. Sometimes, the child can massage his or her own body parts throughout the day. A clever teacher used a pump bottle of lotion that the children could use to massage their hands in preparation for handwriting. Another teacher encouraged children to rub their hands together with lotion to help themselves calm and reduce undesirable behaviors.

It often is difficult to massage the arms when the child is learning to grasp, transfer, and play with toys. An alternative is to do the upper-extremity massage in prone if the child is simultaneously developing weight bearing on the forearms or hands.

1. Symmetrical Starting Stroke

This is a simultaneous stroking of the arms from the shoulder to the hand.

This may be the only stroke that children with extreme upper-extremity sensitivity can tolerate without an increase in tone or behavioral irritability. This is an excellent starting point for providing additional tactile input to the arms.

The stroke

1. Stroke both arms simultaneously from the tops of the shoulders to the hands.

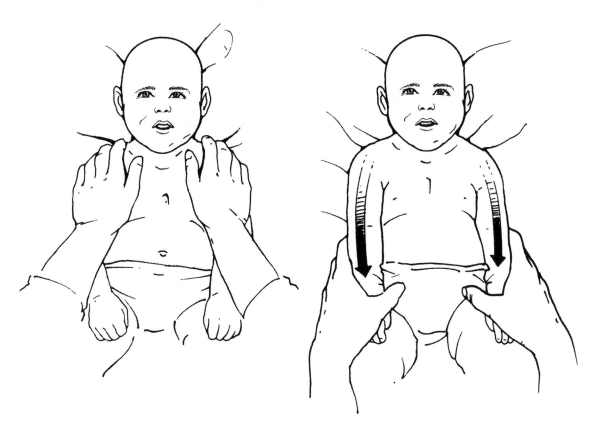

2. Move one hand to the child's shoulder while maintaining contact with your other hand at the child's hand. Then return your other hand to the shoulder.

3. Repeat.

Clinical Implications—This stroke provides symmetrical midline tactile input emphasizing both upper extremities to come forward. This is an excellent stroke for children who rarely get their hands to midline. It is beneficial to children with hypertonicity and those with hypotonicity in their shoulder girdle.

2. Indian Milking—Away From the Heart

Apply firm but gentle pressure from the shoulder to the hand, alternating strokes between the inner (medial) and outer (lateral) aspect of the extremity.

The stroke

1. Support the arm at the inside wrist with one hand. Stroke the arm from the outer border of the shoulder to the wrist.

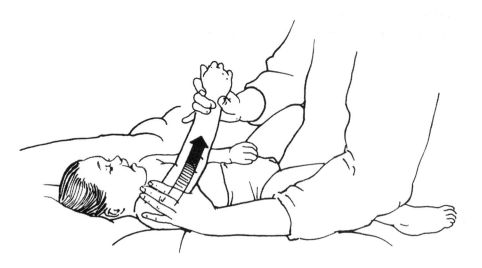

2. Alternate your hands. Start at the inner part of the shoulder and stroke to the wrist.

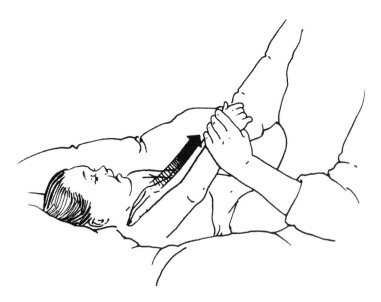

3. Continue to alternate inner and outer strokes, moving from the shoulder to the wrist.

Clinical Implications—As with the leg strokes, this stroke proceeds in a proximal to distal direction. The stroke goes with the pattern of hair growth, facilitating relaxation of tone when performed in a smooth, rhythmical manner. This stroke is very relaxing for most children and often assists in gaining improved range of motion at the shoulder girdle. The authors emphasize active attempts at reaching to midline or for the lower extremities during this stroke. The child also may want to reach for the massage-giver's face. Many reaching activities can be incorporated easily into this stroke.

3. Wringing

This is a gentle squeeze-and-twist motion from the shoulder to the wrist.

The stroke

1. Wrap your hands around the upper arm.

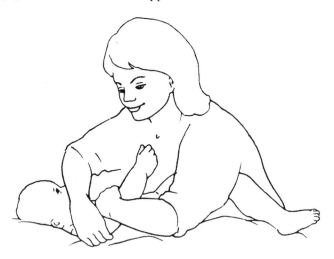

2. Gently wring the arm in both directions by twisting your hands together and then apart, gliding from the shoulder to the wrist.

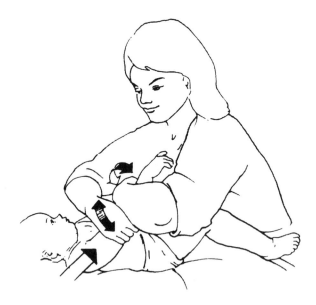

3. As your hands come to the wrist, bring one hand back to the shoulder, then follow with the other. This assures consistent contact.

4. Repeat.

Clinical Implications—As with the leg strokes, this incorporates slight cross friction that gently compresses muscle/connective tissue against bone. This may be difficult for the child with hypersensitivity to tolerate; first massage less sensitive areas to prepare the child. Lubrication is required due to the high level of friction. This stroke may assist in mobilizing the soft tissues of the biceps, triceps, and forearm musculature. It is an excellent method to prepare the forearm for mobilization and subsequent hand expansion.

4. Thumb Press in Palm

This stroke is a maintained pressure into the palms.

The stroke

Press your thumbs into the pads of the palm under the thumb and little finger. Maintain pressure for at least 3 to 5 seconds.

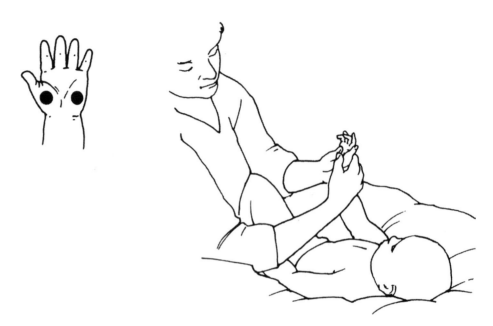

Clinical Implications—This stroke is useful for children with predominant fisting/retention of grasp reflex. The goal is to achieve hand-opening. It is important to maintain the integrity of the hand arches while providing pressure. It also is important to elongate the web space, as you are doing this stroke to preserve opposition in the hand.

5. Small Circles in Palm

In this stroke pressure is applied in a circular motion into the palm.

This stroke may be stimulating and is most appropriate for the child with normal or low-muscle tone in the hand.

The stroke

1. Using your thumbs, make circles in the palm of the hand.

2. Move your thumbs to a new location in the palm and make circles.

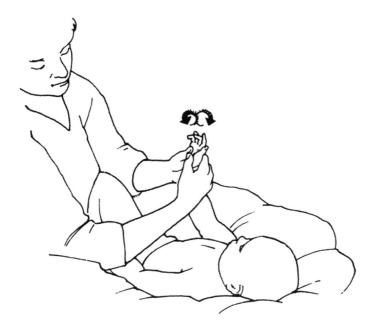

Clinical Implications—This stroke is helpful in activating the intrinsic muscles of the hand as a preparation for hand function. It is important to promote neutral alignment at the wrist and provide contour to the hand. A working knowledge of the palmar (transverse, longitudinal, and oblique) arches is helpful in providing this stroke.

6. Squeeze Each Finger

This stroke is a squeezing and rolling of the fingers.

The stroke

1. Gently grasp the base of the thumb (on the top and bottom surface) between your thumb and index finger.

2. Slide your fingers from the base to the tip of the thumb. Use a gentle, rolling, squeezing motion.

3. Repeat with each finger in order.

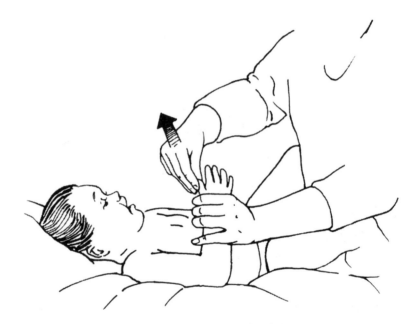

Clinical Implications—This is a good time to talk or sing songs about the fingers and hands. Be aware of joint laxity; do not provide undue traction (gentle pulling). Visual contact with the hand and the fingers is encouraged with songs and finger plays. It is important that the wrist be in a neutral position or in slight extension to achieve full elongation of the long finger flexors, if tightness exists. If the hand is very tightly fisted, simply hold it between your relaxed hands.

7. Stroke Top of Hand

This is a stroking of the back of the hand from the fingers to mid-forearm.

If holding the hand at the palm and backside causes increased flexor tone in the child with hypertonicity, provide a stable point of contact at the sides of the hand or wrist.

The stroke

1. Use your flattened fingers to stroke the top of the hand from the fingers to approximately mid-forearm.

2. Repeat.

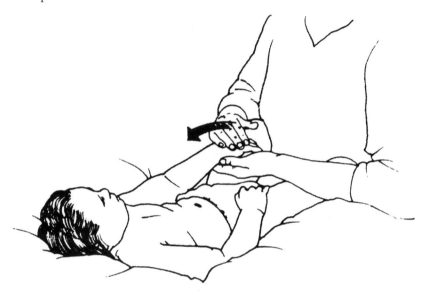

Clinical Implications—The goals are to achieve hand opening and emphasize active wrist extension, which is important in functional grasp.

8. Circles Around the Wrist

This is a continuous stroke around the wrist similar to *Circles Around the Ankles.*

The stroke

1. Move your index and middle fingers simultaneously in a circle around the wrist bones (the ulnar and radial styloid processes). This also may be done with your thumbs.

2. Continue the circular motion.

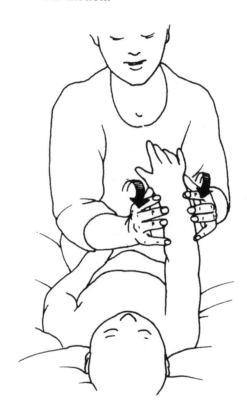

Clinical Implications—The bony prominences around the wrist often are very sensitive in some children. If the child is required to wear hard splints, this area may be even more sensitive. This stroke may help prevent skin breakdown in conjunction with a properly fitted hand splint.

9. Swedish Milking—Toward the Heart

Apply firm but gentle pressure from the hand to the shoulder with lighter pressure when returning to the hand. Alternate the hands between the inner (medial) and outer (lateral) aspects of the extremity.

The stroke

1. Support the arm with one hand at the inside wrist. Use your other hand to stroke firmly from the wrist to the shoulder on the outside surface of the arm.

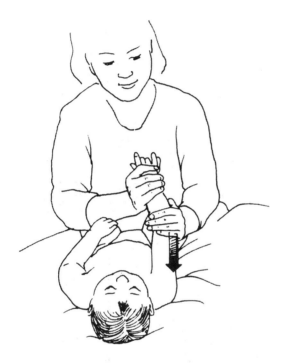

2. Stroke around the shoulder without breaking contact.

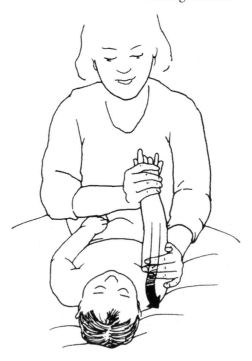

3. Stroke back toward the wrist using your finger pads and a lighter pressure.

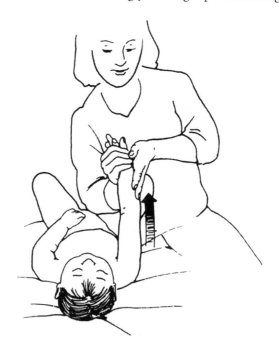

4. Switch hands by supporting the arm at the outside wrist. Use the palm of the other hand to stroke firmly from the inside wrist to the shoulder girdle.

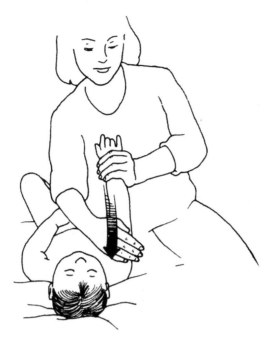

5. Stroke back toward the wrist using your finger pads and a lighter pressure.

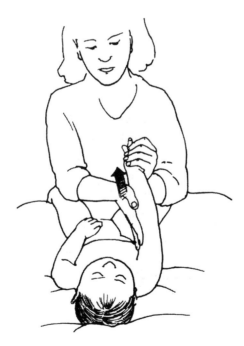

6. Repeat. Continue alternating hands.

Clinical Implications—This stroke emphasizes firm but gentle pressure from the hand to the shoulder with lighter pressure when returning to the hand. Hands alternate between inner (*medial*) and outer (*lateral*) aspects of the extremity. This stroke emphasizes directional pressure moving toward the heart. Swedish massage strokes are slightly more stimulating; they may be used therapeutically with the child with low tone and/or lethargy, to produce arousal. It also is therapeutic for the child with high tone. You may incorporate range of motion throughout the stroking to gain increased range at the shoulder girdle. Elongation of the pectoral muscles may be accomplished as the hand glides down the medial border of the arm, while scapular mobility may be emphasized on the downward portion of the lateral border of the arm. Scapulo-humeral and scapulo-thoracic mobility also can be achieved. This is important for functional reach and shoulder-girdle mobility.

Because of direction and alternating pressures, the strokes may overstimulate the sensitive child. Introduce excitatory strokes gradually and balance them with relaxing strokes (such as Indian Milking).

10. Rolling

This is a gentle, rolling finishing stroke from the shoulder to the wrist.

The stroke

1. Cup your hands around the child's upper arm.

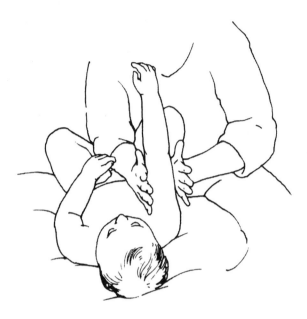

2. Gently alternate your hands to produce a rolling motion (like rolling dough). Simultaneously glide your hands toward the wrist while rolling.

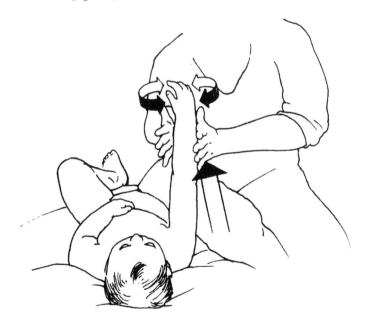

3. When your hands reach the wrist, pause a moment to enable the child to accommodate to the input before repeating the stroke.

4. To ensure continued contact, maintain one hand at the wrist while moving the other hand to the upper arm.

5. Repeat.

Clinical Implications—This is a gentle, rolling finishing stroke from the shoulder to the wrist. It may overstimulate the sensitive child. You may combine it with language sounds to enhance the playful effect of this brisk stroke. This is an ideal time to encourage the child to communicate more, either through sign or verbal language. This stroke may be combined with slight traction to activate musculature at the shoulder girdle.

If this stroke is too stimulating, use a gentle patting on the arm for relaxation. To decrease the stimulation even further, simply place your hands firmly but gently around the upper arm. Maintain this position for at least 3 seconds before moving your hands to a new location closer to the wrist. Cover the entire area for the most complete sensation.

Back

Most children enjoy and benefit from strokes to the back. The child is generally placed in prone over the massage-giver's lap for the back massage. (For additional positioning options, see Chapter 11).

Several precautions apply to back massage:

- Be careful not to apply undue pressure directly to the vertebral column.

- Do not stroke against the pattern of hair whorls—this could be disorganizing for the child.

- Avoid the back of the neck if touch to this area produces undesirable extension.

- If the child cannot comfortably be positioned in prone, use alternative positioning.

1. Swooping to the Bottom

This is a gentle stroking motion from the neck to the buttocks.

Cup your hand so that pressure is applied to the muscles along the spine (the *paravertebral musculature*) and not to the spine. If possible, remove the child's diaper to allow for a more even stroke and sensation. Be careful not to increase pressure at the lower back, as this may cause increased swayback (*lordosis*).

The stroke

1. Place one hand under the child's buttocks as a contact point.

2. Cup the other hand and glide it from the neck, down the middle of the back to the buttocks.

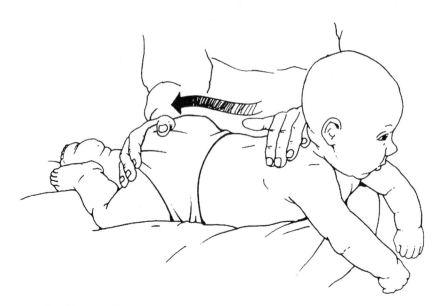

3. Return the stroking hand to the neck and repeat.

Clinical Implications— This stroke usually is applied with slow, rhythmical, even pressure and goes in the direction of hair growth; it tends to provide relaxation. Begin this stroke at the top of the head, if the child enjoys tactile input to the area and if stroking over the back of the neck does not produce undesirable extension. Beginning at the head may enhance body scheme by enabling the child to feel the connection between the head, neck, and back. Use gentle pressure if massaging over the head, avoiding the infant's fontanel's (*soft spot*).

2. Swooping to the Ankles

This is the same as *Swooping to the Bottom*, but the stroke continues to the ankles.

The stroke

1. Support the legs by holding the ankles with one hand. This will establish a point of contact.

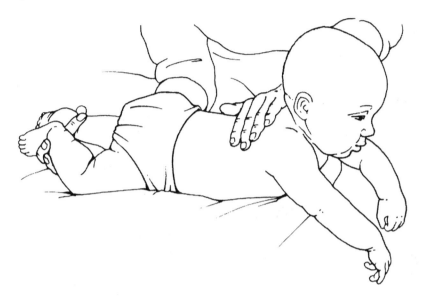

2. Stroke from the neck (or head) to the feet using your other hand.

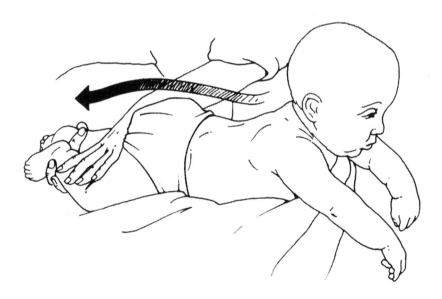

3. Repeat.

Clinical Implications—This stroke may enhance body scheme by giving the child a feeling of connection between the head or neck, the trunk, and the legs To avoid increasing lordosis (*arching*), do not lift the legs when positioning the child for this stroke. For larger children, it may be necessary to stroke from the neck and down one leg. The next stroke would follow with the other leg.

3. Back and Forth

In this stroke hands move back and forth as you proceed up and down the back.

This stroke is relaxing for most children.

The stroke

1. Place your relaxed hands at the shoulders.

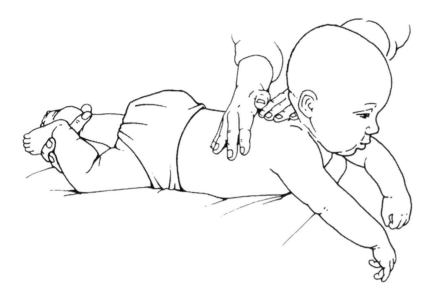

2. Alternate your hands back and forth, gliding over the entire back surface from the shoulders to the buttocks.

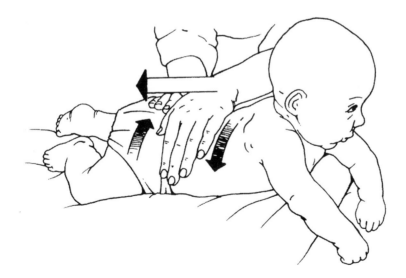

3. Return gliding hands back and forth from the buttocks to the shoulders.

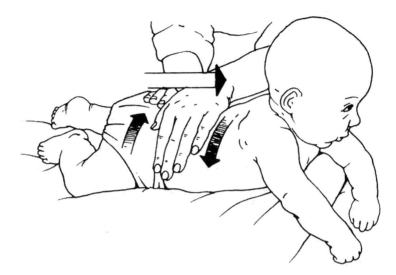

Clinical Implications—This stroke provides an excellent opportunity to assist in shaping the torso. Many children present with flattening of the torso or flaring of the ribs. This flaring may be due to inactive oblique abdominals in combination with limited movement. This stroke may be provided to lift up the lateral borders of the trunk, and may be combined with lateral weight shifting in prone.

4. Small Circles All Over the Back

This stroke incorporates small clockwise circles over the paravertebral area.

It focuses on the muscles along the spine (paravertebral muscles) and not on the vertebral column.

The stroke

1. Place your finger pads together on one side of the base of the spine.

2. Moving your hands in unison, make clockwise circles that move up to the top of the spine.

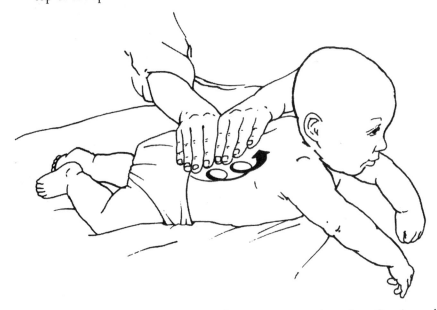

3. Cross over to the other side, avoiding pressure on the spine. Continue the circular motion down to the bottom of the spine.

4. Cross again to the other side and repeat.

Clinical Implications—This stroke may be too stimulating for some children, especially if done too quickly. To downgrade the input, move your hands very slowly and rhythmically. This stroke also may be done with the whole hand and cover a larger surface area, such as for the older child.

5. Combing

This stroke is a vibrating motion proceeding from the top of the spine to the buttocks. Use it as a finishing stroke for the back sequence.

The stroke

1. Place one hand on the nearest hip or shoulder as a maintained point of contact.

2. Shape your hand like a comb and place it on the top of the spine near the shoulder.

3. Gently vibrate your hand from side to side while moving from the top of the spine to the buttocks.

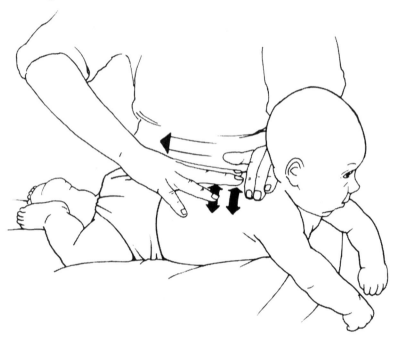

4. Repeat, making each stroke lighter and lighter. End with a feather-light touch.

Clinical Implications—Use your whole hand if the child is overly sensitive to this stroke. Slowly vibrate your hand as it moves from top to bottom, maintaining an even pressure throughout the stroke. You may begin with firmer pressure and, with each successive stroke, get lighter with your touch. Another alternative is very slow even pressure down the spine.

Face

Be sure to respect the child's degree of acceptance of facial touching. Even some children and adults with normally functioning neurological systems do not like to have their faces massaged. Also, children with past or current respiratory concerns are rightfully protective of their airway. Strokes around the nose or mouth may produce anxiety that works against the purpose of the massage. Try to keep your thumbs tucked in, so that they do not block the child's vision or airway.

Do not use oil for the face massage. There is sufficient natural oil on the face, and you risk getting oil or lotion in the child's eyes.

These strokes are specifically designed to proceed toward midline to promote lip closure. Be sure to maintain midline alignment of the head with a neutral chin tuck when you present oral strokes. It also may be necessary to control the jaw when working toward lip closure.

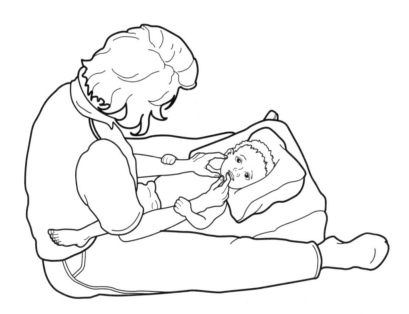

1. Forehead to Mouth

This is a symmetrical stroking from the forehead over the cheeks to the mouth.

The stroke

1. Place the finger pads of both hands at the middle of the child's forehead.

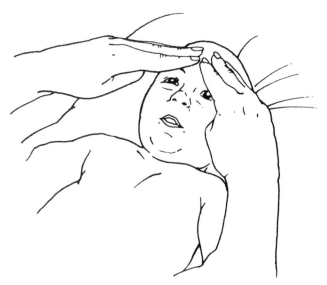

2. Move your hands out and downward over the cheeks, bringing them back together near the mouth.

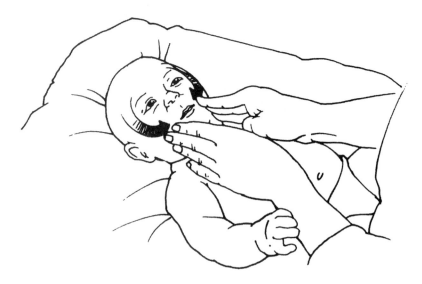

3. Repeat.

Clinical Implications—This stroke elongates the frontalis or forehead muscle, which can collect a good deal of tension with stress; thus, this stroke tends to be relaxing.

2. Eyebrows to Mouth

This is a symmetrical stroking from the eyebrows to the mouth.

The stroke

1. Place the finger pads of both hands at midline, eyebrow level.

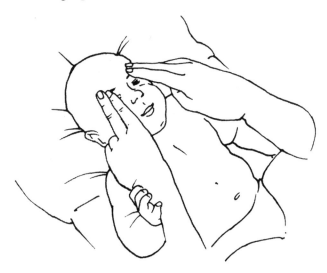

2. Move your hands out and downward over the cheeks, bringing them back together near the mouth.

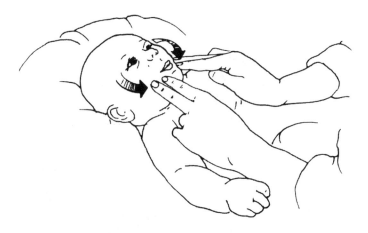

3. Repeat.

Clinical Implications—This stroke is an adaptation of adult massage techniques to relieve sinus pressure. It also assists the cheeks and lips to come to a neutral position when the jaw is in neutral alignment.

3. Nose to Mouth

This is a symmetrical stroking from the sides of the nose to the mouth.

The stroke

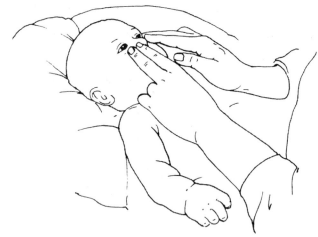

1. Place your finger pads on both sides of the nose.

2. Move your hands out and downward over the cheeks, bringing them back together near the mouth.

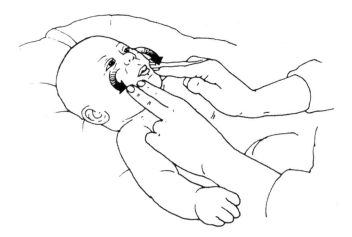

Clinical Implications—This stroke helps achieve cheek and lip alignment when the jaw is in neutral alignment. It soothes some children with nasal congestion.

4. Pressure Toward the Mouth

This entails small strokes with maintained pressure toward the mouth.

The stroke

1. Place the side of your index finger just below the child's nose.

2. Make a small stroke from just below the nose to the lips, encouraging lip closure.

3. Maintain pressure at the lip line for at least 3 to 5 seconds.

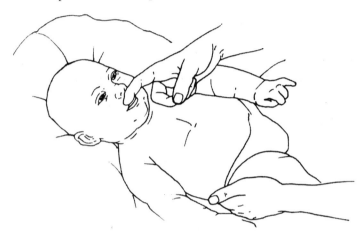

4. Repeat, moving the starting point progressively around the mouth.

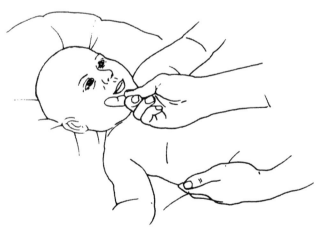

Clinical Implications—This stroke elongates the obicularis oris muscle and works toward proper lip closure. It is helpful to maintain your pressure and move entirely through the range of the lip in a diagonal direction.

5. Finishing Stroke for the Face

This is a stroking from the temple, to behind the ears, and across the cheeks to the mouth.

Some children can tolerate this stroking around the ears even if they have difficulty accepting tactile input to other areas of the face or head.

The stroke

1. Place your finger pads on the child's temples, just above the tops of the ears.

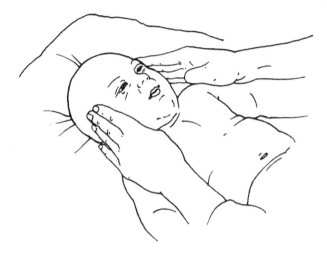

2. Move your hands over and behind the ears.

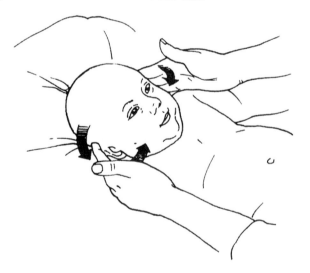

3. Continue across the cheeks to the mouth.

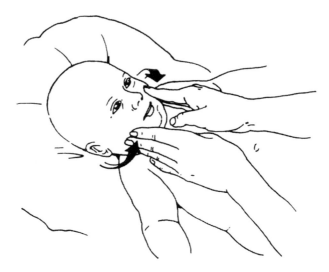

4. Repeat the series. Try to maintain contact with the child's face and head throughout.

Clinical Implications—For children who are very sensitive to touch around the face, this may be the only stroke that is acceptable. You may need to further decrease the input by eliminating step 3. You may be able to start with this stroke and gradually introduce the face strokes that move across the cheeks.

Resources

Here are just a few of many excellent sources of information, education, and supplies for infants' and children's development and massage. This list is solely to help you get started; no endorsement of these products or services is intended or should be inferred.

Information and Training

Our website may be found at **http://www.pediatricmassage.com.** Please refer to this site for updates regarding ongoing workshops and resource/reference material.

Nursing Child Assessment Satellite Training (NCAST)
> CDMRC, Res. 110, WJ-10
> University of Washington
> Seattle, WA 98195
> Phone: 206-543-8528
>
> Offers a variety of programs and assessments for professionals working with families with children under three years of age as well as parent booklets. Programs include information regarding sleep; infant state, behavior, and cues; state modulation; and feeding interaction. Videotape programs and assessment tools include *Keys to Caregiving, Community Health Care Assessments,* and *Parent-Child Interaction Feeding and Teaching Scales.*

Infant Behavioral Assessment and Intervention Program
> Rodd Hedlund, M.Ed.
> Clinical Instructor of Pediatrics/Neonatology
> Infant Development Specialist
> Oklahoma Infant Transition Program
> Sooner NIDCAP® Training Center
> University of Oklahoma Health Sciences Center
> Children's Hospital of Oklahoma
> 4B 4402
> 940 NE 13th Street
> Oklahoma City, Oklahoma 73104
> Phone: 405-271-6625
> Email: rodd-hedlund@ouhsc.edu

Offers education and training for Early Intervention Professionals in:

1. The Infant Behavioral Assessment (IBA)
2. The Neurobehavioral Curriculum for Early Intervention (NCEI)
3. Holding Parents Holding Their Baby

Newborn Individualized Developmental Care and Assessment Program (NIDCAP)
Dr. Heidelise Als
National NIDCAP Training Center Director
Neurobehavioral Infant and Child Studies Laboratories
Children's Hospital
Enders Pediatric Research Building
320 Longwood Avenue, EN-107
Boston, MA 02115
Phone: 617-355-8249

Provides information regarding training in the NIDCAP (a structured observation of the infant's behavioral repertoire and development of individual caregiving recommendations.)

The Brazelton Institute
1295 Boylston Street
Suite 320
Boston, MA 02115
Phone: 617-355-4959
FAX: 617-859-7215
Website: http://web1.tch.harvard.edu/brazelton

Offers training in the use of the Brazelton Neonatal Behavioral Assessment Scale, books, videos, and newsletter.

Touch Research Institute
Department of Pediatrics (D-820)
University of Miami School of Medicine
P.O. Box 016820
Miami, FL 33101
Website: http://www.miami.edu/touch-research

Provides training and ongoing research regarding touch and massage. Website has an extensive summary of research projects. Offers a newsletter and annual symposium.

International Association of Infant Massage Instructors (IAIMI), Inc.
1891 Goodyear Avenue, Suite 622
Ventura, CA 93003
Phone: 805-644-8524
FAX: 805-644-7699
Email: IAIM4US@aol.com
Website: www.iaim-us.com

Provides infant massage instructor training, information, and resources.

Foundation for Healthy Family Living
Kalena Babeshoff, Founder
PO. Box 1665
Sonoma, CA 95476
Phone: 707-996-3545
FAX: 707-996-7187
Website: www.healthyfamily.org

Provides infant massage training, educational materials, information, and resources that enhance respectful communication and nurturing touch.

Parent Tools Educational Warehouse and Infant Massage Programs
Maria Mathias, BA, LMT
605 Bledsoe NW
Albuquerque, NM 87107
Phone: 505-341-9381
Website: www.infantmassageprograms.com

Offers infant massage instructor training and continuing education, as well as books, videos, and educational materials.

Supplies, Books, and Music

IAIM "Gentle Touch" Educational Warehouse, Inc.
1891 Goodyear Avenue
Suite 622
Ventura, CA 93003-8001
Phone: 805-644-9272 or 888-448-9489
FAX: 805-644-7699
Email: gtw4us@aol.com
Website: http://www.iaim-us.com

Carries supplies for infant massage including oil, books, videotapes on infant massage, audiocassettes (relaxation music, lullabies), dolls, and back-supporting floor chairs.

Zenith Supplies
6300 Roosevelt Way N.E.
Seattle, WA 98115
Phone: 206-525-7997 or 1-800-735-7217
Website: www.zenithsupplies.com

Offers therapeutic products including massage oils and lotions, essential oils, massagers, and bolsters for positioning. Zenith also carries books on therapeutic massage for adults.

Steven Halpern's Inner Peace Music
222 Van Tassel Court
San Anselmo, CA 94960
Phone: 1-800-909-0707

FAX: 415-485-1312

Website: www.stevenhalpern.com

"Music for health, relaxation and pure listening pleasure." Publishes a catalog of CD's, audiocassettes, and videotapes.

Discovery Toys, Inc.

P.O. Box 5023

Livermore, CA 94551-5023

Phone: 1-800-426-4777

Website: www.discoverytoysinc.com

Check with your local Discovery Toys educational consultant. The selection "Lullaby Magic" by Joanie Bartels is excellent. It also is available at some card shops. "Sounds Like Fun" is a good choice for more stimulating music.

Also check local stores for quieting or stimulating music, depending on the needs of the child and your personal preference.

Understanding My Signals

By Brenda Hussey-Gardner, Ph.D., M.P.H.

Copyright 1988, 1996

Available through VORT Corporation

P.O. Box 60132

Palo Alto, CA 94306

Photo booklet for parents of preterm infants. Describes infants' approach signals, coping signals, avoidance signals, and strategies to enhance interaction.

Young Living Essential Oils

250 South Main Street

Payson, UT 84651

Phone: 1-800-763-9963

Website: www.youngliving.com

Offers essential and massage oils, and educational books and tapes.

Biotone

4757 Old Cliffs Road

San Diego, CA 92120

1-800-445-6457

FAX: 1-800-664-7567

Website: www.biotone.com

Offers massage oils and lotions, musical selections, and educational videotapes.

You also may want to check local health food stores, massage therapy schools, and on-line booksellers (e.g., amazon.com) for massage oils, lotions, books, videos, music, and other products.

References

Bonding/Attachment

Anderson, G. (1991). Current knowledge about skin to skin-kangaroo care for preterm infants. *Journal of Perinatology, 11,* 216–226.

Gill, B. (1997). *Changed by a child: Companion notes for parents of a child with a disability.* New York: Doubleday.

Kerr, T. (1999). Do kids communicate better with Dad than Mom? *ADVANCE for Occupational Therapy Practitioners, 6,* 12–34.

Klaus, M., & Fanaroff, A. (1986). *Care of the high-risk neonate.* Philadelphia, PA: W.B. Saunders.

Klaus, M. & Kennel, J. (1982). *Parent-infant bonding* (2nd ed.). St. Louis: C.V. Mosby.

Klaus, M., Kennel, J., & Klaus, P. (1995). *Bonding: Building the foundations of secure attachment and independence.* Reading, MA: Addison-Wesley.

Klaus, M., & Robertson, M. (Eds.). (1982). *Birth, interaction, and attachment.* Skillman, NJ: Johnson & Johnson Baby Products.

Kubler-Ross, E. (1993). *On death and dying.* New York: Maxwell MacMillan.

McCroskey, K. (1989). On Mother's Day and finally home. *Baby Talk, 5,* 32–33.

Nelson, D. (1994). *Compassionate touch: Hands-on caregiving for the elderly, the ill and the dying.* Barrytown, NY: Station Hill Press.

Perske, R. (1981). *Hope for the families: New directions for parents of persons with retardation or other disabilities.* Nashville, TN: Abingdon Press.

Reite, M. (1984). Touch, attachment, and health–is there a relationship? In C. C. Brown (Ed.), *The many facets of touch.* Skillman, NJ: Johnson & Johnson Baby Products.

Winnicott, D. W. (1987). *Babies and their mothers.* Beverly, MA: Addison-Wesley.

The High-Need Baby

DeGangi, G. (1991). Assessment of sensory, emotional, and attentional problems in regulatory disordered infants. Part 1. *Infants and Young Children, 3,* 1–8.

DeGangi, G., Craft, P., & Castellan, J. (1991). Treatment of sensory, emotional and attentional problems in regulatory disordered infants. Part 2. *Infants and Young Children, 3,* 9–19.

Jones, S. (1992). *Crying baby, sleepless nights* (Rev. ed.). Boston, MA: Harvard Common Press.

Scheider, P. (1989). *Parents' book of infant colic.* New York: Ballantine Books.

Sears, W. (1984). *The fussy baby.* New York: New American Library.

Sears, W. (1991). *Keys to calming the fussy baby.* New York: Barrens Educational Series.

Sears, W., & Sears, M. (1996). *Parenting the fussy baby and high need child.* New York: Little, Brown and Company.

Spock, B. (1987). *Babies and their mothers.* Beverly, MA: Addison Wesley.

Infant Massage

Auckett, A. (1981). *Baby Massage.* New York: Newmarket Press.

Cady, S. H., & Jones, G. E. (1997). Massage therapy as a workplace intervention for reduction of stress. *Perceptual and Motor Skills, 84,* 157–158.

Drehobl, K., & Fuhr, M. (1988). Infant massage helps parents interact with newborn. *OT Week, 42*(2), 5.

Drehobl, K., & Fuhr, M. (1988). A neurophysiological approach to infant massage. *OT Forum, 44*(3), 1–7.

Drehobl, K., & Fuhr, M. (1991). *Pediatric massage for the child with special needs.* Tucson, AZ: Therapy Skill Builders.

Fuhr, M. (1987). Massage for infants and young children. *OT Forum, 43*(2), 1–6.

Heinl, T. (1982). *The baby massage book.* Englewood Cliffs, NJ: Prentice Hall.

LeBoyer, F. (1976). *Loving hands.* New York: Alfred Knopf.

Longworth, J. C. B. (1982). Psychophysiological effects of slow stroke back massage in normotensive females. *Nursing Science, 4*(44), 44–61.

McClure, V. (1988). *Infant massage instructor's manual.* Portland, OR: International Association of Infant Massage Instructors.

Ohashi, W. (1986). *Touch for love.* New York: Ballantine Books.

Porter, S. (1996). The use of massge for neonates requiring special care. *Complimentary Therapies in Nursing & Midwifery, 2,* 93–96.

Rice, R. (1978). *The loving touch book.* Dallas: Cradle Care.

Rush, A. (1989). *The back rub book.* New York: Vintage Books.

Schneider, E. F. (1999). *Touch communication: The power of infant massage.* Foundation for Healthy Living [On-line news posting]. URL http://www.healthyfamily.org/new.html

Schneider, V. (1982). *Infant massage: A handbook for loving parents.* New York: Bantam Books.

Schneider, V. (1988). *Infant massage instructors manual.* United States Publication.

Schneider-McClure, V. (1989). *Infant massage: A handbook for loving parents* (Rev. ed.). New York: Bantam Books.

Sinclair, M. (1992). *Massage for healthier children.* Oakland, CA: Wingbow Press.

Speirer, J., Garty, M., Miller, K., & Martinez, B. *Infant massage for developmentally delayed babies.* Denver, CO: United Cerebral Palsy Center.

Thomas, S. (1988). *Massage for common ailments.* New York: Simon and Schuster.

Walker, P. (1987). *Baby relax.* New York: Pantheon Books.

Walker, P. (1988). *The book of baby massage.* New York: Simon and Schuster.

Walker, P. (1988). Special handling. *Parenting Magazine, 10,* 88–92.

Walker, P. (1995). *Baby massage: A practical guide to massage and movement for babies and infants.* New York: St. Martin's Press.

Development/Medicine/Neurophysiology

Als, H. (1986). A synactive model of neonatal behavioral organization: Framework for the assessment and support of the neurobehavioral development of the premature infant and his parents in the environment of the neonatal intensive care unit. *Physical and Occupational Therapy in Pediatrics, 6,* 3–55.

Als, H. (1992). Individualized, family-focused developmental care for the very low birthweight preterm infant in the NICU. In S. L. Freidman and M. D. Sigman (Eds.), *The psychological development of low birthweight children* (pp. 341–388). Norwood, NJ: Ablex.

Als, H. (1997). Earliest intervention for preterm infants in the newborn intensive care unit. In M. J. Guralnick (Ed.), *The effectiveness of early intervention* (pp. 47–76). Baltimore: Paul Brooks.

Als, H. & Gilkerson, L. (1997). The role of relationship-based developmentally supportive newborn intensive care in strengthening outcome of preterm infants. Seminars in Perinatology, 21(3), 178–189.

Als, H., Lester, B., Tronick, E., & Brazelton, T. (1982). Toward a research instrument for the assessment of preterm infants' behavior. In H. Fitzgerald, B. Lester, and M. Yogman (Eds.), *In theory and research in behavioral pediatrics* (pp. 1, 35–63). New York: Plenum Press.

American College of Neuropsychopharmacology. (1988). Need for mother's touch is brain based. *Science, 239,* 142–143.

Autism Society of America home page (1999, October). [WWW document]. URL http://www.autism-society.org/

Barnard, K. (1987). *Nursing child assessment feeding scale.* Seattle: NCAST Publications.

Barnard, K. (1989). *Nursing child assessment satellite training learning resource manual.* Seattle: NCAST Publications.

Barr, H., & Kiernan, J. (1983). *The human nervous system.* Philadelphia, PA: Harper and Row.

Behrman, R. (1994). *Nelson essentials of pediatrics.* Philadelphia. W. B. Saunders.

Bennett, F. C. (1990). Recent advances in developmental intervention for biologically vulnerable infants. *Infants and Young Children, 3*(1), 33–40.

Biel, A. (1997). *Trail guide to the body.* Boulder, CO: Andrew Biel, LMP.

Blackburn, S. (1989). Sleep and awake states of the newborn. In K. E. Barnard (Ed.), *Nursing child assessment satellite training resource manual.* Seattle: NCAST Publications.

Blackburn, S. (1978). *Early parent-infant relationships.* White Plains, NY: March of Dimes Defects Foundation.

Bly, L. (1983). *The components of normal movement during the first year of life and abnormal motor development.* Oak Park, IL: Neurodevelopmental Therapy Association.

Bly, L. (1991). A historical and current view of the basis of NDT. *Pediatric Physical Therapy, 3*(3), 131–136.

Bly, L. (1994). *Motor skills acquisition in the first year of life.* Tucson, AZ: Therapy Skill Builders.

Bly, L., & Whiteside, A. (1997). *Faciliation techniques based on NDT principles.* San Antonio, TX: Therapy Skill Builders.

Boehme, R. (1988). *Improving upper body control: An approach to assessment and treatment of tonal dysfunction.* Tucson, AZ: Therapy Skill Builders.

Brazelton, T. (1984). *Neonatal behavior assessment scale.* Philadelphia: J. B. Lippencott.

Brodal, P. (1998). *The central nervous system structure and function* (2nd ed.). New York. Oxford University Press.

Brown, D. (1980). *Neurosciences for allied health therapies.* St. Louis, MO: C. V. Mosby

Browne, J. V., VandenBerg, K., Ross, E. S., & Elmore, A. M. (1999). The newborn developmental specialist: Definition, qualifications and preparation for an emerging role in the neonatal intensive care unit. *Infants and Young Children, 11*(4), 53–64.

Calais-Germain, B. (1993). *Anatomy of movement.* Seattle, Washington: Eastland Press.

Calkins, S. D. (1997). Cardiac vagal tone indices of temperamental reactivity and behavioral regulation in young children. *Developmental Psychology, 31,* 125–135.

Cannon, W. B. (1939). *The wisdom of the body* (2nd ed.). New York: Norton Publishing.

Clayman, C. (Ed.). (1989). *The American Medical Association encyclopedia of medicine.* New York: Random House.

Corff., K., Seideman., R., Venkataraman, S., Lutes., L., & Yates, B. (1995). Facilitated tucking: A nonpharmoacologic comfort maeasure for pain in preterm neonates. *Journal of Obstetrical and Gynecological Nursing, 2,* 143–147.

DeGangi, G. (1994). *Documenting sensorimotor progress: A pediatric therapist's guide.* Tucson, AZ: Therapy Skill Builders.

Dorland's illustrated medical dictionary. (1974). Philadelphia: W.B. Saunders.

Ericks, J. (1989). *Infant talk. Nursing child assessment satellite training learning resource manual.* Seattle: NCAST Publications.

Farber, S. (1982). *Neurorehabilitation: A multi-sensory approach.* Philadelphia: W.B. Saunders.

Field, T. (1990). *Infancy.* Cambridge, MA: Harvard University Press.

Field, T. (Ed.). (1995). *Touch in early development.* Mahwah, NJ: Lawrence Erlbaum Associates.

Fraiberg, S. (1987). The origins of human bonds. In L. Fraiberg (Ed.), Selected writings of Selma Fraiberg (pp. 1–26). Columbus: Ohio State University Press.

Frank, L. K. (1971). *Tactile communication, NCB Kopp: Reading in early development for occupational and physical therapy students.* Springfield, IL: Charles C. Thomas.

Geldard, F. A. (1972). *The human senses* (2nd ed.). New York: John Wiley and Sons.

Gellhorn, E. (1967). *Principles of autonomic-somatic integration.* Minneapolis: University of Minnesota Press.

Gunzenhauser, N. (1987). *Infant stimulation: For whom, what kind, when, and how much?* Skillman, NJ: Johnson and Johnson Baby Products.

Gunzenhauser, N. (1990). *Advances in touch: New implications in human development.* Skillman, NJ: Johnson and Johnson Consumer Products.

Guyton, A. (1981). *Basic human neurophysiology.* Philadelphia: W.B. Saunders.

Harrell, L. (1984). *Touch the baby. Blind and visually impaired children as patients: Helping them respond to care.* New York: American Foundation for the Blind.

Hedlund, R. (1989). Fostering positive social interactions between parents and infants. *Teaching Exceptional Children, Summer,* 45–48.

Hedlund, R. (1996). *The neurobehavioral curriculum for early intervention.* Publication available from Washington Research Institute, 150 Nickerson Street, Suite 305, Seattle, WA 98104.

Hedlund, R., & Tatarka, M. (1988). *The Infant Behavioral Assessment.* Publication available from Experimental Education Unit, CDMRC, WJ-10, University of Washington, Seattle, WA 98195.

Holloway, E. (1998). *Relationship-based occupational therapy in the neonatal intensive care unit* (2nd ed.). Pediatric Occupational Therapy and Early Intervention. Boston: Butterworth-Heinemann.

Holmes, J., & Lindsley, D. (1984). *Basic human neurophysiology.* New York: Elsevier.

Huffman, L. C., Bryan, Y. E., del Carmen, R., Pederson, F. A., Doussard-Roosevelt, J. A., & Porges, S. W. (1995). Infant temperament and cardiac vagal tone: Assessments at twelve weeks of age. *Child Development, 69*(3), 624–635.

Huss, A. (1977). Touch with care or a caring touch? *American Journal of Occupational Therapy, 31*(1), 11–18.

Hussey-Gardner, B. (1996). *Understanding my signals: Help for parents of premature infants.* Palo Alto, CA: VORT Corporation.

Hyde, A., & Trautman, S. (1989). Drug-exposed infants and sensory integration: Is there a connection? *American Occupational Therapy Association, 12*(4), 1–6.

Ironson, C. (1996). Fragile creations, therapists foster developmentally appropriate care for premature infants. *PT and OT Today, October,* 18–21.

Izard, C. E., Porges, S. W., Simons, R. F., Haynes, O. M., & Cohen, B. (1991). Infant cardiac activity: Developmental changes and relations with attachment. *Developmental Psychology, 27*(3), 432–439.

Kandell, E., Schwartz, J., & Jessel, T. (1991). *Principles of neural science* (3rd ed.). Norwalk, CT: Appleton and Lange.

Krupp, M., & Chatton, M. (Eds.). (1981). *Current medical diagnosis and treatment.* Los Altos, CA: Lange Medical Publications.

Lawhon, G. (1997). Providing developmentally supportive care in the newborn intensive care unit: An evolving challenge. *Journal of Perinatal Neonatal Nursing, 10*(4), 48–61.

Lewis, K., & Thomson, H. (1986). *Manual of school health.* Menlo Park, CA: Addison-Wesley.

Littel, E. (1990). *Basic neuroscience for the health professions.* Thoroughfare, NJ: Slack.

Miller, M. Q., & Quinn-Hurst, M. (1994). Neurobehavioral assessment of high-risk infants in the neonatal intensive care unit. *The American Journal of Occupational Therapy, 48*(6), 506–513.

Modrcin-McCarthy, M., Harris, M., & Marlar, C. (1997). Touch and the fragile infant: comparison of touch techniques with implications for nursing practice. *Mother Baby Journal, 2*(4), 12–19.

Molnar, G. (Ed.). (1985). *Pediatric rehabilitation.* Baltimore: Williams and Wilkins.

Moran, M., Radzyminski, S., Higgins, K., Dowliing, D., Miller M., & Cranston-Anderson, J. (1999). Maternal kangaroo (skin to skin) care in the NICU beginning 4 hours postbirth. *Maternal Child Nursing, 24*(2), 74–79.

Nelson, W., Behrman, R., Kliegman, R., & Arvin, A. (Eds.). (1996). *Nelson textbook of pediatrics* (15th ed.). Philadelphia, PA: W.B. Saunders.

Neu, M., & Voyles-Brown, J. (1997). Infant physiologic and behavioral organization during swaddled versus unswaddled weighing. *Journal of Perinatology 17*(3), 193–198.

Noback, C., & Demarest, R. (1977). *The nervous system.* New York: McGraw Hill.

Oski, F. (1989). *Principles and practice of pediatrics.* Philadelphia: J.B. Lippincott.

Pansky, B. (1988). *Review of neuroscience* (2nd ed.). New York: Macmillan.

Peele, T. L. (1977). *The neuroanatomic basis for clinical neurology* (3rd ed.). New York: McGraw Hill.

Powley, T. (1999). Central control of autonomic functions: The organization of the autonomic nervous system. In M. Zigmond, F. Bloom, S. Landis, J. Roberts, and L. Squire (Eds.) Fundamental Neuroscience. San Diego, CA: Academic Press.

Ryder, R. (1988). Management of patient/therapist via employment sensorimotor approach. *OT Forum, 22,* 7–9.

Sach, F. (1988). The intimate sense. *Sciences, 1,* 28–34.

Seidel, H., Ball J., Dains J., & Benedict G. W. (1999). *Mosby's guide to physical examination* (4th ed.). Portland: Mosby.

Semmler, C., & Hunter, J. (1990). *Early occupational therapy intervention.* Gaithersburg, MD: Aspen Publications.

Sweeney, J. (Ed.). (1986). *The high-risk neonate: Developmental therapy perspectives.* New York: Hayworth Press.

Trombley, C., & Scott, A. (1977). *Occupational therapy for physical dysfunction.* Baltimore: Williams and Wilkins.

Umphred, D. (1985). *Neurological rehabilitation.* St. Louis, MO: Mosby Publications.

University of Washington School of Nursing. (1989). *State-related behaviors and individual differences. Nursing child assessment satellite training resource manual.* Seattle: NCAST Publications.

VandenBerg, K. (1990). Behaviorally supportive care for the extremely premature infant. In Gunderson and Kenner (Eds.), *Small baby protocol care of 24–25 week infants.* Petaluma, CA: Neonatal Network Publications.

VandenBerg, K. (1993). Basic competencies of begin developmental care in the intensive care nursery. *Infants and Young Children, 6*(2), 52–59.

VandenBerg, K. & Franck, L. (1990). Behavioral issues for infants with BPD. In C. Llund (Ed.), *BPD strategies for total patient care*. Petaluma, CA: Neonatal Network Publications.

Walton, T. (1998). Contraindications to massasge therapy, roadblocks on the way to consensus. *Massage Therapy Journal, 37*(2) 108–112.

Walton, T. (1999). Contraindications to massage, taking a history. *Massage Therapy Journal, 37*(4), 70–92.

Whiteside, A. (1997). Clinical goals and application of NDT facilitation. *NDTA Network, September,* 1–14.

Zigmond, M., Bloom, F., Landis, S., Roberts, J., & Squire, L. (1999). *Fundamental neuroscience.* San Diego, CA: Academic Press.

Research

Acolet, D., Modi, N., Giannakoulopoulos, X., Bond, C., Weg, W., Clow, A., & Glover, V. (1993). Changes in plasma cortisol and catecholamine concentrations in response to massage in preterm infants. *Archives of Disease in Childhood, 68,* 29–31.

Anderson, G., Marks, E., & Wahlberg, V. (1986). Kangaroo care for premature infants. *American Journal of Nursing, 7,* 806–807.

Barnard, K., Booth, C., & Johnson-Crowley, N. (1985). Infant massage and exercise: Worth the effort? *Mother Child Nurse, 3,* 184–189.

Clark, O., & Ensher, G. (1986). *Newborns at risk.* Gaithersburg, MD: Aspen Publications.

Cullen C., Field, T., Hernadez-Reif, M., Field., T., Sprinz, P., & Beebe, K. (in preparation). *Pediatric oncology patients benefits from massage therapy.* [On-line news posting]. URL http://www.miami.edu.touch.research.

Deiter, J., Field, T., & Hernadez-Reif, M. (in preparation). *Prostate cancer symptoms are reduced by massage therapy.* [On-line news posting]. URL http://www.miami.edu.touch.research.

Dossetor, D. R., Couryer, S., & Nichol, A. R. (1991). Massage for very severe self-injurious behavior in a girl with Cornelia de Lange syndrome. *Developmental Medicine and Child Neurology, 33*(7), 636–640.

Fernandez, A., Patkar, S., Chawla, C., Taskar, T., & Prabhu, S. (1987). Oil application in preterm babies: A source of warmth and nutrition. *Indian Pediatrics, 24,* 1111–1116.

Field, T. (1980). Supplemental stimulation of preterm neonates. *Early Human Development, 4*(3), 301–314.

Field, T. (1995). Massage therapy for infants and children. *Journal of Developmental & Behavioral Pediatrics, 16*(2), 105–111.

Field, T. (1998). Massage therapy effects. *American Psychologist, 53*(12), 1270–1281.

Field, T., Grizzle, N., Scafidi, F., Abrams, S., & Richardson, S. (1996). Massage therapy for infants of depressed mothers. *Infant Behavior and Development, 19*, 109–114.

Field, T., Grizzle, N., Scafidi, F., & Schanberg, S. (1996). Massage and relaxation therapies' effects on depressed adolescent mothers. *Adolescence, 31*(124), 903–911.

Field, T., Henteleff, T., Hernandez-Reif, M., Martinez, E., Mavunda, K., Kuhn, C., & Schanberg, S. (1998). Children with asthma have improved pulmonary functions after massage therapy. *Journal of Pediatrics, 132*(5), 854–858.

Field, T., Hernandez-Reif, M., LaGreca, A., Shaw, K., Schanberg, S., & Kuhn, C. (1997). Massage therapy lowers blood glucose levels in children with Diabetes Mellitus. *Diabetes Spectrum, 10*, 237–239.

Field, T., Hernadez-Reif, M., Quintino, O., Schanberg, S., & Kuhn C. (1998). Elder retired volunteers benefit from giving massage therapy to infants. *Journal of Applied Gerontology, 17*, 229–239

Field, T., Hernandez-Reif, M., Seligman, S., Krasnegor, J., Sunshine, W., Rivas-Chacon, R., Schanberg, S., & Kuhn, C. (1997). Juvenile rheumatoid arthritis: Benefits from massage therapy. *Journal of Pediatric Psycholgy, 22*(5), 607–617.

Field, T., Ironson, G., Scafidi, F., Nawrocki, T., Goncalves, A., Burman, I., Pickens, J., Fox, N., Schanberg, S., & Kuhn, C. (1996). Massage therapy reduces anxiety and enhances EEG pattern of alertness and math computations. *Journal of Neuroscience, 86*, 197–205.

Field, T., Kilmer, T. Hernandez-Reif, M., & Burman, I. (1996). Preschool children's sleep and wake behavior: Effects of massage therapy. *Early Child Development and Care, 120*, 39–44.

Field, T., Lang, C., Martinez, A., Yando, R., Pickens, J., & Bendell, D. (1996). Preschool follow-up of infants of dysphoric mothers. *Journal of Clinical Child Psychology, 25*(3), 272–279.

Field, T., Lasko, D., Mundy, P., Henteleff, T., Kabat, S., Talpins, S., & Dowling, M. (1997). Brief report: Autistic children's attentiveness and responsivity improve after touch therapy. *Journal of Autism and Developmental Disorders, 27*(3), 333–338.

Field, T., Lasko, D., Mundy, P., Henteleff, T., Talpins, S., & Dowling, M. (1996). Autistic children's attentiveness and responsivity improved after touch therapy. *Journal of Autism and Developmental Disorders, 27*, 329–334.

Field, T., Morrow, C., Valdeon, C., Larson, S., Kuhn, C., & Schanberg, S. (1992). Massage reduces anxiety in child and adolescent psychiatric patients. *Journal of the American Academy of Child & Adolescent Psychiatry, 31*(1), 125–131.

Field, T., Peck, M., Krugman, S., Tuchel, T., Schanberg, S., Kuhn, C., & Burman, I. (1998). Burn injuries benefit from massage therapy. *Journal of Burn Care & Rehabilitation, 19*(3), 241–244.

Field, T., Quintino, O., Hernandez-Reif, M., & Koslovsky, G. (1998). Adolescents with attention deficit hyperactivity disorder benefit from massage therapy. *Adolescence, 33*(129), 103–108.

Field, T., Scafidi, F., & Schanberg, S. (1987). Massage of preterm infants to improve growth and development. *Pediatric Nursing, 13*(6), 385–386.

Field, T., Schanberg, S., Kuhn, C., Fierro, K., Henteleff, T., Mueller, C., Yando, R., Shaw, S., & Burman, I. (1998). Bulimic adolescents benefit from massage therapy. *Adolescence, 33*(131), 555–563.

Field, T., Schanberg, S., Scafidi, F., Bauer, C., Vega-Lahr, N., Garcia, R., Nystrom, J., & Kuhn, C. (1986). Tactile/kinesthetic stimulation effects on preterm neonates. *Pediatrics, 77*(5), 654–658.

Field, T., Seligman, S., Scafidi, F., & Schanberg, S. (1996). Alleviating posttraumatic stress in children following Hurricane Andrew. *Journal of Applied Developmental Psychology, 17*(1), 37–50.

Hansen, R., & Ulrey, G. (1988). Motorically impaired infants: Impact of a massage procedure on caregiver-infant interactions. *Journal of the Multihandicapped Person, 1*(1), 61–68.

Harrison, L., Leeper, J. & Yoon, M. (1990). Effects of early parent touch on preterm infants' heart reates and arterial oxygen saturation levels. *Journal of Advanced Nursing, 15*, 877–885.

Harrison, L., Ollivet, L., Cunningham, K., Bodin, M., & Hicks, C. (1996). Effects of gentle human touch on preterm infants: pilot study results. *Neonatal Network, 15*(2), 35–42.

Hernandez-Reif, M., Field, T., Krasnegor, J., Martinez, E., Schwartzman, M., & Mavunda, K. (1999). Children with cystic fibrosis benefit from massage therapy. *Journal of Pediatric Psychology, 24*, 175–181.

Jay, S. (1982). The effects of gentle human touch on mechanically ventilated very-short-gestation infants. *Maternal Child Nursing Journal, 11*(4), 199–257.

Knaster, M. (1998). Tiffany Field provides proof positive. *Massage Therapy Journal, 37*(1), 84–88.

Korner, A., & Schneider, P. (1983). Effects of vestibular-proprioceptive stimulation of neurobehavioral development of preterm infants: A pilot study. *Neuropediatrics, 14,* 170–175.

Kramer, M., Chamorro, I., Green, D., & Knudtson, F. (1975). Extra tactile stimulation of the premature infant. *Nursing Research, 24*(5), 324–334.

Krug, D., Arick, J., & Almond, P. (1979). Autism screening instrument for educational planning: Background and development. In J. Gillum (Ed.), *Autism diagnosis, instruction, management and research.* Austin, TX: University of Texas Press.

Nelson, D., Heitman, R., & Jennings, C. (1986). Effects of tactile stimulation on premature infant weight gain. *Journal of Obstetric, Gynecologic, and Neonatal Nursing, 3,* 262–267.

Oehler, J. (1985). Examining the issue of tactile stimulation for preterm infants. *Neonatal Network, 12,* 25–33.

Pardew, E. M. (1996). The effects of infant massage on the interactions between high risk infants and their caregivers (Doctoral dissertation, Oregon State University, 1996). *Dissertation Abstracts International, 18,* 9634072.

Portela, A. (1990). Massage as a stimulation technique for premature infants: An annotated bibliography. *Pediatric Physical Therapy, 2*(1), 80–85.

Rausch, P. (1981). Effects of tactile and kinesthetic stimulation on premature infants. *Journal of Obstetric, Gynecologic, and Neonatal Nursing, 10*(1), 34–37.

Rice, R. (1977). Neurophysiological development in premature infants following stimulation. *Developmental Psychology, 13*(1) 7–26.

Rice, R. (1979). Effects of the Rice infant sensorimotor stimulation treatment on the development of high-risk infants. *Birth Defects: Original Article Series, 15*(7), 69–76.

Ross, E. (1984). Review and critique of research on the use of tactile and kinesthetic stimulation with premature infants. *Physical and Occupational Therapy in Pediatrics, 1,* 35–49.

Saigal, S., & Whyte, R. (1987). Tactile/kinesthetic effects on preterm neonates. *Pediatrics, 79*(1), 165–166.

Scafidi, F., & Field, T. (1996). Massage therapy improves behavior in neonates born to HIV-positive mothers. *Journal of Pediatric Psychology, 21*(6), 889–897.

Scafidi, F., Field, T., & Schanberg, S. (1990). Massage stimulates growth in preterm infants: A replication. *Infant Behavior and Development, 13*(2), 167–188.

Scafidi, F., Field, T., Schanberg, S., Bauer, C., Tucci, K., Roberts, J., Morrow, C., Kuhn, C. (1990). Massage stimulates growth in preterm infants: A replication. *Infant Behavior and Development, 13*(2), 167–188.

Scarr-Salapatec, S., & Williams, M. (1972). A stimulation program for low birth weight infants. *American Journal of Public Health, 62*(5), 662–667.

Schachner, L., Field, T., Hernandez-Reif, M., Duarte, A. M., & Krasnegor, J. (1998). Atopic dermatitis symptoms decreased in children following massage therapy. *Pediatric Dermatology, 15*(5), 390–395.

Scholtz, K., & Samuels, C. (1992). Neonatal bathing and massage intervention with fathers, behavioral effects 12 weeks after birth of the first baby: The Sunraysia Australia Intervention Project. *International Journal of Behavioral Development, 15*(1), 67–81.

Seibert, J., Hogan, A., & Mundy, P. (1982). Assessing interactional competencies: The early social-communication scales. *Infant Mental Health Journal, 3*, 244–245.

Strong, C. (1989). The effect of massage on premature infants. Doctoral dissertation, University of Arizona, College of Nursing, (1989). *Dissertation Abstracts International,* 9000148.

Verhoef, M. J., & Page, S. A. (1998). Physicians' perspectives on massage therapy. *Canadian Family Physician, 44*, 1018–1024.

White, J., & Labarba, R. (1976). The effects of tactile and kinesthetic stimulation on neonatal development in the premature infant. *Developmental Psychobiology, 9*(6), 569–577.

White-Traut, R., & Goldman, M. B. (1988). Premature infant massage: Is it safe? *Pediatric Nursing, 11*(4), 285–289.

White-Traut, R., & Nelson, M. (1988). Maternally administered tactile, auditory, visual, and vestibular stimulation: Relationship to later interactions between mothers and premature infants. *Research in Nursing and Health, 11*, 31–39.

White-Traut, R., & Pate, C. (1987). Maternally administered tactile, auditory, visual, and vestibular stimulation: Relationship to later interactions between mothers and premature infants. *Research in Nursing and Health, 11,* 31–39.

White-Traut, R., & Tubeszewski, K. (1986). Multimodal stimulation of the premature infant. *Journal of Pediatric Nursing, 1*(2), 90–95.

Sensory Integration

Ayres, A. J. (1973). *Sensory integration and learning disorders.* Los Angeles: Western Psychological Services.

Ayres, A. J. (1979). *Sensory integration and the child.* Los Angeles: Western Psychological Services.

Fisher, A., Murray E., & Bundy, A. (1991). *Sensory integration, theory and practice.* Philadelphia, PA: F. A. Davis.

Kranowitz C. (1998). *The out of sync child.* New York: Skylight Press.

Miller, L., & Kinnealey, M. (1999). *Researching the effectiveness of sensory integration.* Sensory Integration Resource Center [On-line news posting]. URL http://www.sinetwork.org/Articles/researching_the_effectiveness_of_si/cover_research_effectiveness.htm

Royeen, C. & Lane, S. (1991). Tactile processing and sensory defensiveness. In A. Fischer, E. Murray, & A. Bundy (Eds.) *Sensory integration theory and practice.* Philadelphia, PA: FA Davis.

Wilbarger, J., & Stackhouse, T. (1999). *Sensory modulation: A review of the literature.* Sensory Integration Resource Center [On-line news posting]. URL http://www.sinetwork.org/Articles/SM_-_Review_of_OT_Literature/sensory_modulation_ot_lit_review.htm

Wilbarger P., & Wilbarger, J. (1991). Sensory defensiveness definition http://www.sinetwork.org/Articles/SM_-_Review_of_OT_Literature/wilbarger__wilbarger_copy(1).htm

Wilbarger, P., & Wilbarger, J. (1995). Class notes from Treatment for Sensory Defensiveness.

Tactile Intervention/Massage

Alva, M. (1999). Getting in touch with children: Pediatric massage can help parents relax and communicate with youngsters who have special needs. *ADVANCE for Speech-Language Pathologists and Audiologists, 3,* 26.

Alva, M. (1999). Hands on love. *ADVANCE for Physical Therapists and PT Assistants, 2,* 50.

Anderson, J. (1986). Sensory intervention with the preterm infant in the neonatal intensive care unit. *The American Journal of Occupational Therapy, 4*(1), 19–25.

Baranek, G. T., Foster, L. G., & Berkson, G. (1997). Tactile defensiveness and stereo-typed behaviors. *The American Journal of Occupational Therapy, 51*(2), 91–95.

Beck, M. (1988). *The theory and practice of therapeutic massage.* New York: Milady Publishing Corp.

Beck, M. (1994). *Milady's theory and practice of therapeutic massage* (2nd ed.). Albany, NY: Milady Publishing.

Brown, C., Barnard, K., & Brazelton, T. (Eds.). (1984). *The many facets of touch.* Skillman, NJ: Johnson & Johnson Baby Products.

Cohen, S. (1987). *The magic of touch.* New York: Harper and Row.

Colton, H. (1983). *Touch therapy.* New York: Kensington Publishing.

Elliott, M. (1999). *Cancer fighters: Congressional hearings focus on alternative treatments.* Massage & Bodywork [On-line news posting]. URL http://www.softlineweb.com/

Feeny, T. (1995). Hands-on therapy: Touching lives of children through pediatric mas-sage. *ADVANCE for Physical Therapists, 6*(9), 8–9.

Feltman, J. (Ed.). (1989). *Hands-on healing.* Emmaus, PA: Rodale Press.

Fritz, S. (1995). *Mosby's fundamental of therapeutic massage.* St. Louis, MO. Mosby-Year Book.

Fritz, S., & Mosby Editorial Board. (1996). *Mosby's visual guide to massage essentials.* St. Louis, MO. Mosby-Year Book.

Guyer, E. (1992). *From the hand to the heart.* New York: Author.

Holloway, E. (1987). Critically ill, full-term infant . . . lacks sensory input of others. *OT Week, 7*(2), 4–5.

Hosler, R. (1982). *Massage book.* Mountain View, CA: Runner's World Books.

Juhan, D. (1998). *Job's body.* Barrytown, NY: Station Hill Openings.

Krieger, D. (1975). Therapeutic touch: The imprimatur of nursing. *American Journal of Nursing, 75*(5), 784–787.

Kulka, A., Fry, C., & Goldstein, G. (1960). Kinesthetic needs in infancy. American *Journal of Orthopsychiatry, 30,* 562–571.

Landsmann, M. (1999). Healing hands: Science of touch. *ADVANCE for Directors in Rehabilitation, 8*(6), 45–49.

Lidell, L., Thomas, S., Cooke, C., & Porter, A. (1984). *The book of massage.* New York: Simon & Schuster.

Lowe, W. (1997). *Functional assessment in massage therapy* (3rd ed.). Bend, OR: Orthopedic Massage Education and Research Institute.

McCormack, G. (1991). *Therapeutic use of touch.* Tucson, AZ: Therapy Skill Builders.

Miller, E. (1999). *Intervene early with infant massage.* The Gentle Touch Program [On-line news posting]. URL http://main.nc.us/gentletouch/ARTICLES-6-Intervene_Early.html

Montague, A. (1986). *Touching: The human significance of the skin* (3rd ed.). New York: Harper and Row.

Nelson, D. (1994). *Compassionate touch: Hands-on caregiving for the elderly, the ill and the dying.* Barrytown, NY: Station Hill Press.

Newton, D. (1998). *The clinical pathology for the professional bodyworker.* Portland, OR: Simran Publications.

Rattray, F. (1994). *Massage therapy: An approach to treatments.* Toronto, Ontario: Massage Therapy Texts and MAVerick Consultants.

Robbins, G., Powers, D., & Burgess, S. (1994). *A wellness way of life* (2nd ed.). Madison, WI: Brown & Benchmark.

Sinclair, A. (1999). *Adapting infant massage for older children.* Internet Magazine [On-line news posting]. URL http://www.suite101.com/article.cfm/infant_massage/12827

St. John, J. (1987). *High tech touch: Acupressure in the schools.* Novato, CA: Academic Therapy Publications.

Tappan, F. (1988). *Healing massage techniques.* East Norwalk, CT: Appleton and Lange.

Tappan, F. (1998). *Tappan's handbook of healing massage techniques.* Stanford, CT. Appleton and Lange.

Wall, A. (1998). Baby massage: probably of benefit. *Professional care of mother and child, 8*(4), 86.

Weiss, S. (1979). The language of touch. *Nursing Research, 28*(2), 76–80.

Werner, R., & Benjamin, B. (1998). *A massage therapist's guide to pathology.* Baltimore, MD: Williams and Wilkins.

Wood, E., & Becker, P. (1981). *Beard's massage.* Philadelphia: W.B. Saunders.